When Survival Became a Choice

My Family's Journey Through Cancer — and the Path Back to Health

Elena Rybak

Published by Living Healthy Institute

The information presented in this book reflects the author's personal experiences and professional perspectives and is intended for educational purposes only. It is not intended to replace professional medical advice, diagnosis, or treatment. Readers should always consult qualified healthcare professionals regarding medical conditions or treatment decisions.

The author and publisher assume no responsibility for any adverse effects resulting from the use of the information contained in this book.

First Edition

Dedication

For Manuel —
for your strength, resilience,
and the courage with which you chose to keep fighting.

For our sons —
whose love gave this fight its deepest purpose.

You carried your own battles through these years.
May life guide each of you toward strength, purpose, and peace.

A Note to the Reader

This book tells the story of a very personal journey through illness, survival, and the search for healing.

What you will read here is not only the experience of a family facing cancer, but also the perspective of someone who has spent more than twenty years as a holistic health practitioner.

Throughout this journey we combined conventional medical treatment with nutritional, environmental, emotional, and lifestyle-based support strategies.

The ideas and practices described in these pages come from lived experience, years of professional practice, and ongoing research and observation.

This first part is the story — what happened and how we made decisions in real time.

In Part 2, I explain in detail the therapies, supplements and approaches we used — what they are, why we chose them, and how they work.

Every person, every body, and every illness is different. Nothing in this book is meant to replace medical care or professional advice. Instead, it is offered as a story, a perspective, and a collection of tools that guided us through one of the most difficult chapters of our lives.

My hope is that the experiences shared here may provide insight, encouragement, or simply a sense that no one walks this path alone.

Contents

Chapter 1 — The Day Everything Changed 7

Chapter 2 — Snow and Normal Life............................16

Chapter 3 — Looking for Answers 23

Chapter 4 — Understanding...28

Chapter 5 — The Plan 33

Chapter 6 — Hospital 38

Chapter 7 — Diagnosis..43

Chapter 8 — The First Round.......................................49

Chapter 9 — The Fight 53

Chapter 10 — The Other Battles 60

Chapter 11 — The Angel in the Sky 63

Chapter 12 — The Final Shot 66

Chapter 13 — Chemo Brain 71

Chapter 14 — Living Through the Battle 75

Chapter 15 — Another Scare 79

Chapter 16 — When the War Ends...............................84

Chapter 17 — What the War Taught Me.......................91

Chapter 18 — Foundation of Healing 99

Chapter 19 — Therapeutic Nutrition During Crisis.......107

Chapter 20 — Parasites, Internal Terrain, and Hidden Burdens.......120

Chapter 21 — Supplement Strategy and Rotations.....132

Chapter 22 — The Nervous System, Emotions, and the Body's Ability to Heal.......138

Chapter 23 — The Life After.......145

About the Author.......152

Chapter 1 — The Day Everything Changed

"Elena..."

The moment I heard his voice, my stomach dropped.

Instead of saying hello, the words came out of my mouth before I even thought about them.

"It can't be good."

There was a short pause on the other end of the phone.

"No," he said quietly. "It is not."

My heart started pounding.

"What you and I felt earlier," he continued, "was just the tiny tip of a very large iceberg."

Another pause.

"The mass is the size of a mango."

The room began to spin.

I slowly slid down the wall until I was sitting on the floor.

A mango.

My brain tried to process the words but couldn't quite catch up.

"Is it cancer?" I asked.

"Most likely"

"The radiologist was almost sure of it. They just didn't know what kind yet. He suspected lymphoma."

I thanked him for calling, hung up the phone, and sat there on the floor.

The tears came immediately.

From the living room I could hear laughter.

My two youngest boys were climbing all over their dad on the couch. Five and two years old, completely unaware that their world had just changed.

My thoughts raced faster than I had ever experienced before.

Will he die?
How soon?
Will they remember him?
How am I going to raise these boys alone?

I had done it once before. I had been a single mom to my oldest son until he was nine years old. Then Manuel came into our lives and everything changed.

Now my boys were
Fifteen,
Five and
Two.

They needed their father.

The first person I called was my mom.

The moment she heard my voice she started crying. I almost never cried in front of her, so she knew something terrible had happened.

"Manuel likely has cancer," I said through sobs.

That was all I knew.

And now I had to go tell him.

I hung up the phone and sat there for another minute, trying to gather myself.

Crying wasn't an option right now.

Not in front of the kids.

I went to the bathroom, washed my face, and looked at myself in the mirror.

Then I walked back into the living room.

My legs felt strangely disconnected from the rest of my body.

Manuel looked up at me from the couch. The boys were still climbing on him like a jungle gym.
He studied my face for just a moment.

"It's bad, huh?"

I nodded.

He didn't ask anything else.

He just kept playing with the kids, smiling at them like nothing had happened.

That was Manuel.

Even then, he was protecting them.

Later that night, after the boys were finally asleep, we sat down together.

I told him what little I knew.

A large mass. Almost certainly cancer. Possibly lymphoma.

He listened quietly.

Then he looked straight at me.

"Now what?"

His eyes were full of something I will never forget.
Hope.

Complete belief that I would know what to do.

Do I? Me?

By that time I had been a holistic practitioner for seventeen years. I had worked with many people. I had seen incredible recoveries. I had guided people through all kinds of health challenges.

But those were their stories.

Not mine.

Not my husband.

People came to me for guidance—cleansing protocols, diet advice, supplements, lifestyle changes. Sometimes they had very serious illnesses. Even cancer.

But it was always their journey.

I was someone standing on the outside trying to help.

Now the man I loved, the man I had chosen to build my life with, was sitting in front of me asking what we were going to do about cancer.

We had only been together six years.

Six years.

What kind of cruel test was this?

For a moment I felt fear rise inside me like a wave.

But then something unexpected happened.

The way he looked at me—with so much trust, so much confidence—gave me strength.

In that moment I made a decision.

Not out loud at first.

Inside.

I chose.

I chose for him to live.

The fear that had been gripping my chest loosened.

I looked at him and said the words with more certainty than I actually felt.

"We are going to beat this."

"We are not going to let some disease take you away from this family."

"We'll figure it out. Step by step."

There was one thing I knew for sure.

Cancer gives time.

It's not a heart attack.
It's not a stroke.

Cancer gives time.

And time means options.

Solutions.

We just had to use that time wisely.

We also made another decision that night.

The younger boys would not know anything.

They were too little to carry that kind of fear. Only our teenager would know, because he would notice something was wrong.

That night I barely slept.

My mind raced through everything I had learned in seventeen years of practice—cleansing protocols, diet, supplements, stories of people who recovered from things doctors said were impossible.

But this time it wasn't a client.

It was my husband.

The man my children called Papi.
The truth was, I didn't know exactly what we were going to do yet.

But I knew one thing with absolute certainty.
Every problem has a solution.

And most of the time, there is more than one.

We just had to find ours.

What made it even harder was something I understood immediately, even if no one said it out loud.

Everyone would be looking at me.

Not just as a wife. Not just as the person holding the family together, paying the bills, caring for the kids.

Something much heavier than that.

Manuel had placed his life in my hands.

He trusted that I would make the decisions. That I would search, research, choose the path, try the treatments, ask the questions doctors might not think to ask.

And that kind of trust comes with a terrifying weight.

Because if he survived, everyone would say we fought well.

But if he didn't?

Then every decision would live with me forever.
Every choice.

Every mistake.

Every path I chose to take — or didn't.

That was the responsibility I felt sitting there in the dark that night.

And there was no way around it.

The only thing I could do was stand up, take it, and move forward.

Because the fight had already begun.

Chapter 2 — Snow and Normal Life

December 2020.
The world was preoccupied with COVID. News, restrictions, masks, fear—everything revolved around it. Travel was complicated, people were canceling plans, staying home, waiting for things to pass.

But we decided to go anyway.

Living in Florida, snow is something magical for us and for the kids. We wanted them to experience a real winter, a real Christmas with snow. So we packed the car and drove to Snowshoe, West Virginia, hoping for that picture-perfect white Christmas.
And we got it.
Cold, snowy, beautiful.

On Christmas Eve a big snowstorm rolled in and covered everything in thick white powder. The mountains looked like something from a postcard.

Our oldest son was skiing.
The middle one was sledding.
And the little one—only two years old—was absolutely terrified of the cold air.

Danny, two, didn't like the way it felt on his face. The air was so crisp and sharp that he would start crying the moment we stepped outside. So Manuel carried him everywhere, wrapped in layers of winter clothes that made him look like a stuffed snowman.

Manuel himself was not exactly a winter expert.

Being from Mexico, he had seen snow only once before in his life. This was only his second time. He kept saying he felt frozen the entire trip, but he was doing his best to enjoy it because the kids were so excited.

We rented a small one-bedroom apartment on the third floor with a beautiful view of the mountain. Manuel and I slept in the bedroom and all three boys slept on air mattresses in the living room.

It was loud.
It was chaotic.
And it was wonderful.

One day the temperature dropped to minus twenty-five degrees. We had tickets for tubing that day. Looking back at the pictures now, we were standing in the snow with our eyelashes literally covered in ice.

Manuel kept carrying Danny everywhere because the little guy refused to walk in the cold. With all the heavy winter clothes—boots, gloves, hats—it wasn't easy. But he did it anyway.

Most of the time we had to take turns. One of us would stay inside with Danny while the other went outside with the older boys. Then we would switch.

It was one of those trips that feels messy and exhausting while you're living it, but later becomes a beautiful family memory.

At least, that's what we thought it would be.

On the last couple of days of the vacation Manuel started saying his stomach hurt.

At first we didn't think much of it. Maybe something he ate. Traveling always changes routines—food, sleep, everything. He said it felt like pulling pressure inside his stomach, but nothing dramatic enough to make us worry.

What I did notice was that he suddenly became very eager to go home.

Normally Manuel is calm and patient about travel. We had driven long distances before and usually broke the trip into two days, stopping at a hotel somewhere along the way.

This time he didn't want that.

"We're going straight home," he said.
I remember looking at him, surprised. Driving from West Virginia back to Florida with three kids in the car is not exactly relaxing.

But he insisted.

So we drove.

We stopped only for gas and quick bathroom breaks. No restaurants, no long stops, no hotel.

Twenty hours in the car.

The car had its own rhythm that day.

Our teenager had his headphones on most of the time, texting friends and disappearing into his music. Every once in a while he would snap and yell at his little brothers to stop screaming.

The five-year-old and I played small games to pass the time—counting cars, spotting license plates from different states, anything to keep him entertained.

And like every parent on a long road trip, we prayed for naps.

When the little ones finally fell asleep the car would go quiet for a while.

But Manuel stayed quiet the entire trip.

That was unusual.

He loves to talk. Normally he would be telling stories, joking with the kids, commenting on the road, the weather, the drivers around us.

This time he barely said anything.

He just drove.

Hour after hour.

His hand resting on his stomach.

And somewhere deep inside me, a quiet voice kept saying that something wasn't right.

The kids were restless. At times the car was loud and chaotic, full of complaints and arguments the way long road trips with children usually are.

When we finally arrived home, I assumed the discomfort would pass once we were back in our normal routine.

But it didn't.
A few days later he developed a fever. No cold symptoms, no cough—just fever and complete exhaustion. For about three days he had almost no energy.

Then it seemed to pass.

Manuel pushed through it the way he always did and said he felt fine again.

He had spent most of his adult life working construction—painting, remodeling, lifting heavy tools and equipment every day. Physical discomfort was not something he usually complained about.

So when the stomach pain returned, we assumed it was something mechanical.

A pulled muscle.
A hernia.
Something from years of lifting heavy things.

At home, once in a while we would dance in the living room.

Tango is how we met.
It's how our relationship began.

That music, the movement, the intensity—tango has a way of pulling two stubborn personalities together.

One evening while lifting me, Manuel suddenly stopped.

A sharp cramp shot through his stomach.

That confirmed our suspicion even more.
"Probably a hernia," we thought.

So we went to see a friend of mine who was a primary care doctor and asked for a referral for a CT scan, just to check.

Manuel was lean, no belly, no extra weight. The doctor pressed on the side where the pain was.

Then he paused.

He said he felt something that didn't quite feel like a hernia.

He asked me to feel it too.

There was a tiny hardness there. Very small. Easy to miss. It could have been nothing, but it was strange enough that the doctor didn't want to ignore it.

So he gave Manuel a referral for a CT scan.

Manuel went straight to the clinic to get it done.

At that moment we still believed we were dealing with something simple.

A pulled muscle.

A hernia.

Something routine.

Cancer was not even a word in our minds yet.

Chapter 3 — Looking for Answers

Manuel came home later that evening just as the scan was finished. And at almost the exact same moment, my phone rang. It was my doctor friend calling from his cell phone.

CT scans don't come back in minutes. Normally it takes days for a radiologist to read the images, send the report, and for the doctor to call with results.

This call came almost immediately.
Before I even answered, I felt my stomach drop.
I stepped into the bedroom to take the call.
Instead of saying hello, the first words out of my mouth were,

"It can't be good."

There was a short pause on the other end.

"No," he said quietly. "It isn't."

He explained that what we had felt during the exam was only a tiny part of something much larger.

"The radiologist says the mass is about the size of a mango."

For a moment everything inside me went still.

He added that the radiologist believed it was most likely lymphoma, although they wouldn't know for certain without further testing.

When I hung up the phone, I sat there for a moment trying to gather myself.

In the living room the kids were still climbing all over Manuel, laughing and asking him to play.

Life in the house was continuing exactly as it had been a few minutes earlier.
But everything had just changed.
That night, after the boys were asleep, Manuel and I talked.
We didn't have answers yet.
Only questions.
But one thing was already clear.
Waiting was not an option.

The next morning life continued as if nothing had happened. Our oldest son went to school. The younger boys were still at home, playing and being boys. Breakfast was made. The house looked exactly the same as it had the day before.

But inside our world was different.
Now we needed answers.
The first question was simple: what exactly were we dealing with?
Normally that answer comes from a biopsy.
But in the world I had worked in for years, biopsies were controversial. Many practitioners believed that puncturing a tumor could break the body's natural containment and allow cancer cells to spread.

Whether that theory was correct or not, it was enough to make us hesitate.

Instead, we decided to begin with another test I knew about — the RGCC test.

It required a blood test that would be sent to a laboratory in Greece. From that blood they could identify circulating tumor cells, determine what type of cancer it might be, and even test which treatments — both pharmaceutical and natural — could potentially work against it.

We agreed to the test. The results would take about three weeks. And three weeks felt like a very long time to sit and do nothing. So we didn't just wait. We worked.
Manuel immediately started an intensive cleansing protocol.

We focused on detoxifying the digestive system, supporting the liver, and stimulating the lymphatic system. At the same time he began a juice fast to give the body a chance to reset and reduce inflammation.

While he worked on his body, I worked on information.
Every free moment I had was spent researching.

During that search I discovered a man named Chris Wark and his website, Chris Beat Cancer. His story and the stories of other survivors were powerful. Chris had survived stage III colon cancer and created a program called Square One — a series of ten one-hour video sessions where he explained everything he had learned during his own fight.

It wasn't just a book or a website.

It was a roadmap.

He talked about diet, supplements, detoxification, and the research behind different approaches. But what struck me most was that he also spoke about something many medical conversations ignore completely — energy, mindset, and spiritual health.

Prayer.

Hope.

The will to live.

Manuel and I watched those videos together.

At that moment we still didn't know exactly what kind of cancer we were dealing with or how aggressive it was. But hearing someone speak calmly and intelligently about surviving cancer changed something inside us.

For the first time since the phone call, the situation didn't feel like a death sentence. It felt like a problem that needed to be solved.

It was from those videos that I first heard about the Hoxsey Biomedical Institute in Mexico.

The Hoxsey clinic had been using a natural cancer protocol for decades. What surprised me most was that patients didn't always need to travel there. They could ship the treatments and guide patients remotely.

I contacted them immediately.

Within a short time we had a consultation scheduled with one of their oncologists. I sent them every piece of medical information we had so far — which honestly wasn't much.

No biopsy yet.
No confirmed diagnosis.

Just the scan and a growing sense that something aggressive was happening inside Manuel's body.

But at least now we were moving.

We had a direction.

And we believed that if we kept searching, we would find the right path.

Chapter 4 — Understanding

After the initial phone call, I barely slept.

My mind was racing — not just as a wife, but as a practitioner.

For seventeen years I had worked with the body from a different perspective than most conventional medical systems. I had always believed that healing does not begin with a diagnosis.

Healing begins with listening.

In my work I had come to understand the body as an intelligent system — constantly processing, adapting, and communicating. Symptoms are not random events. They are signals that something within the system is under strain.

When people talk about "gut health," they often think only about digestion. But in my practice the gut represents something much broader. It is one of the body's central processing centers.

Everything we take in passes through this system.

Food.
Stress.
Thoughts.
Emotions.
Environmental toxins.
Constant stimulation from the modern world.

When the load becomes too heavy, the body does what it is designed to do. It adapts. It stores. It compensates.

Symptoms don't appear because the body is failing, but because it is trying to manage too much.

After Manuel's diagnosis, we began thinking back.

From my own work, and from what we had learned through Chris Wark and many of the survivors he had interviewed, I knew that cancer rarely appears overnight.

It develops over time.

Sometimes the process begins ten years before the first serious symptoms appear.

A single cell mutates — a so-called "mother cell." Instead of dying the way normal cells do, it continues living and replicating.

Why that happens is still not fully understood.

Most likely it is not one single cause, but a combination — a perfect storm.

Parasites.
Fungal infections.
Heavy metals.
Chronic stress.
Unprocessed emotional trauma.
Spiritual Imbalance that goes unseen for years.

All of these can create an internal environment where abnormal cells are able to survive and multiply.

Our internal environment determines far more than we realize.

It influences how we think.
How we feel.
How we digest.
Even how our cells live and die.

Hearing Chris Wark talk about the timeline of cancer was comforting.

If this process had begun years earlier, that meant something important. It meant we still had time to work.

When we looked back, the signs had actually been there.

Two years before the diagnosis, not long after our youngest son was born, Manuel had started experiencing strange symptoms.

Severe anxiety. Episodes of insomnia so intense he could go an entire week barely sleeping at all — yet still somehow function and go to work. His back itched constantly. Sometimes he would stand against the wall just to scratch it for relief.

He tried acupuncture and Chinese herbs, which helped him relax enough to sleep occasionally. But the cycles kept returning. Eventually he even started using Benadryl just to force himself to sleep.

We ran tests. Everything came back normal.

Even earlier than that — about five years before the diagnosis — he had experienced heart palpitations and sudden weight loss. At one point he wore a heart monitor for a week while doctors tried to understand what was happening.

Again, no answers.
Over the years his weight slowly dropped from around 180 pounds to about 156. At the time we didn't connect these events to anything serious. Blood tests were normal. Doctors saw no clear problem. And when there is no diagnosis, it is difficult to know where to look next.

Looking back after the cancer diagnosis, the pattern became much clearer. The body had been trying to communicate with us for years. We simply didn't yet know how to read the signals.

There was one more moment that came back to me during those long nights of thinking.

The day Manuel and I first met.

We met through tango — dancing partners first, then friends, then something much more.
During one of our early conversations he asked about my work. I told him I was a holistic practitioner and that much of my focus was on cleansing the body and restoring balance to the system.

He became curious and scheduled an appointment with me soon after.

He went through a cleansing program and felt significantly better. Digestive issues he had been experiencing disappeared.

He told me that when we met and started talking he had this thought in his head that

"One day this woman is going to save my life."

I just smiled. At that time that message could have meant so many things.

Years later, when my mind was spinning with the weight of decisions I had to make, he reminded me of that moment.

And after everything was over, he reminded me again.

Chapter 5 — The Plan

I started ordering supplements, building a rotation, and planning cleansing protocols. The list was long — too long to use all at once. So I had to think like a strategist.

What mattered most first?

One thing was clear to me: the fight had to come from every direction — physical, emotional, and spiritual. Since we didn't yet know the exact cause, but understood that cancer usually develops from a perfect storm of factors, our response had to address everything.
But there was another realization that became just as important.

I could guide the process.
I could research, plan, and bring the tools.

But I could not fight the battle.

At some point during those weeks I told Manuel something that became our rule for everything that followed.

"I will provide the weapons. But you have to fight."

It may sound simple, but it wasn't. I had seen it many times in my work with people facing serious illness. The moment someone falls into the role of a victim, the fight begins to fade. Fear takes over. Responsibility shifts outward. The body senses that surrender.

That could not happen here.

Manuel could trust me to guide the strategy. He could rely on my knowledge, my research, and my ability to build a plan. But the power had to remain his. His body had to fight. His mind had to choose life. His spirit had to stay engaged.

Without that, no protocol in the world would matter.

So while I ordered supplements, planned cleanses, and searched for answers, he had his role too: to stay mentally present, to participate, and to believe that survival was possible.

From that moment on, we approached everything as a partnership.

I would bring the weapons.
He would fight.

And that's what we began to do.

During those weeks of waiting, I kept coming back to one idea: support the body, don't fight it.

Over time I had come to see that the body is not a machine that suddenly "breaks." It is an intelligent system constantly adapting to what it is given. When the load becomes too heavy — toxins, stress, emotional strain, poor nourishment — the body does what it must to survive. It compensates. It stores. It signals.

Symptoms are not failures of the body. They are messages from a system trying to manage more than it can comfortably carry. What becomes clear when you observe the body long enough is this: the body is almost always working for us, not against us.

When we stop fighting it and begin supporting it, something remarkable often happens. Systems begin to reorganize. Energy returns. Inflammation settles. Clarity improves. The body remembers how to heal.

Healing doesn't come from force. It comes from restoring balance — supporting digestion, detoxification, elimination, nourishment, and immune strength together. The body does not heal in isolated parts. It heals as a whole system.

That understanding shaped every decision I began to make for Manuel. I was not looking for a single miracle cure. I was looking for ways to support the entire system so his body would have the strength to fight — and his spirit would have the will to live.

We started with cleansing.

Before anything else, we needed to clear the body so it can respond. The digestive system, the liver, the lymphatic system — they all play a role in processing and removing waste. If those pathways are overloaded, the body cannot properly absorb the nutrients and support what it needs.

So while we waited for answers, I began preparing the groundwork. This was the work I had been doing for years.

I ordered supplements — some from the United States, others from different parts of the world. Herbs, tinctures, medicinal teas. The list was extensive, but everything had to be carefully rotated so the system would not be overwhelmed.

We scheduled a consultation with the Hoxsey clinic in Mexico for the following week. At that point there was still little they could do without knowing the exact type of cancer, but I wanted every door open.

High-dose Vitamin C IV treatments were also planned at the clinic where the RGCC test had been taken.

But we were still waiting — it felt endless.

I also ordered a book by Louise Hay, *You Can Heal Your Life*. I had already been familiar with her work and had always been fascinated by her as a person — her strength, her philosophy, the way she believed the mind and body were deeply connected.

I ordered the book for Manuel in Spanish. I already had it in English, but I knew that affirmations in his native language would go deeper.

Soon pieces of paper with affirmations were everywhere in our house — on doors, on cabinets, on the bathroom mirror. Every time he passed one, he had to read it.

At first it felt almost silly.

But repetition has power. Eventually those words begin settling into the subconscious.

Prayer also became part of the plan.

Chris Wark had spoken often about faith and the role prayer played in his healing. Manuel's parents were deeply religious and had always prayed regularly, but Manuel and I had never practiced anything structured ourselves.

Still, the idea stayed with him.

Chris had mentioned that not every church carries the same message. Some focus on fear and punishment. Others focus on hope and healing. He suggested finding one that speaks about light.

Manuel decided to try.

He searched for a Spanish-speaking church and went to a service one Sunday.

And on that exact day, during that exact service, the pastor invited a woman to come to the stage and share her daughter's story — a recent cancer survivor.

Manuel later told me his jaw dropped.

This could not be a coincidence. He kept going back. Slowly, his faith began to grow.

Meanwhile, we were still waiting for answers.
On the outside I tried to stay calm and focused.
Inside, every hour felt like a countdown.

Chapter 6 — Hospital

Three weeks later we were called in for the results of the RGCC test.

After all that waiting — and thousands of dollars — the answer was painfully vague. The test confirmed only two things: it was cancer, and it was extremely aggressive. The scale they used went up to five.

Manuel's number was 4.89.

That was it. No type. No direction. Just confirmation that something dangerous was happening.

A couple of days later his condition changed dramatically.

He began vomiting after drinking even small amounts of water. At first we thought maybe his stomach was irritated. But it quickly became clear that something much more serious was happening.

He couldn't keep anything down.

I told him to go to the emergency room and that I would take care of the kids and meet him there. I called my mom and asked her to come stay with them. Picked up my oldest son from school and got everyone settled at home.

Then I rushed to the hospital.

By the time I arrived he had already been admitted. They had taken blood and ordered a CT scan. His condition was deteriorating by the minute. He was vomiting constantly — every few minutes.

His stomach was empty, yet large amounts of liquid kept coming up.

When the scan results returned, the doctors were visibly confused.

What had been described weeks earlier as the size of a mango was now closer to the size of a papaya. It had nearly tripled in size in less than four weeks.

And yet his blood work looked perfect.
The doctors joked that he had the blood of the healthiest 53-year-old in the country. Every marker was normal.
Nothing made sense.

At that point the decision was made to admit him to the hospital. He was too weak to stand, too dehydrated, and vomiting constantly. It was obvious he had cancer, but no one could yet say what kind. The speed of the growth stunned the doctors.

It was the end of February 2021.

COVID was still in full force.

Hospitals were barely allowing visitors. Getting access to him became its own battle. Even when I managed to get upstairs, visiting hours were extremely limited.
Eventually they made me leave, and I had to go home —
but home meant something completely different.

At the hospital I had to stay strong for him. At home I had to stay strong for the rest of my family.

There was no space to fall apart.

I came home, took care of the kids, helped with homework, read bedtime stories, sang songs, and tucked them into bed as if everything was normal.

Only when the house was quiet did I allow myself to break. I went to my room and cried.
Overwhelmed. Exhausted. Terrified. Praying.

The next morning I returned to the hospital. My mom had taken over with the kids.
Inside the hospital, there was nothing to do but wait.

Manuel continued vomiting large amounts of green liquid. He was on IV fluids but could not eat or drink anything. His body rejected everything.

The doctors seemed puzzled. They had theories, but no answers.

They prepared him for two procedures — a biopsy of the mass and a bone marrow biopsy, which were scheduled 3 days out.

Then we waited again. Five days.

Meanwhile doctor after doctor came into the room. Oncologists. Surgeons. Specialists. Each had a different theory.

"If it's this, we'll need to remove these organs."

"If it's that, we'll have to operate immediately."

Some of the scenarios they described sounded brutal — removing large sections of his digestive system, living with permanent bags for bodily functions.

Listening to them slowly eroded my confidence.

Even if they could remove it… what kind of life would that be?

And yet when I looked at Manuel, he kept smiling.

He was weak, skeletal, drifting in and out of sleep, sometimes almost delirious from exhaustion — but every time he saw me, he smiled.

I brought him a Spanish copy of *You Can Heal Your Life*, but he was too weak to hold it.

So I played recordings instead — her lectures and meditations, along with talks by Joe Dispenza. I let them play while he was awake and even while he slept.
I just knew it was important for him to hear those messages.

He continued losing weight rapidly. His body was shrinking in front of my eyes.

And there was something else. A smell.
It is difficult to explain, but some people understand immediately.

Death has a smell.

Not like bad breath or body odor.

Something different.

Something in the air around the person.

I could smell it around him. I knew he was close.
He also strangely calm and peaceful. He kept telling me he felt a presence near him. Maybe it was his guardian angel. But the smell made me feel like death itself was nearby.
Even though my hope for him was still strong, I understood that he was at a crossroads. That things could go either way at any moment.

That was the moment I decided to call his mother.
With my very limited Spanish, I told her she should come. She already knew he was sick. Both she and Manuel's father are deeply faithful people, and they had been praying constantly for their son.

Their attitude and confidence amazed me.

They had complete faith that he would be fine.

No panic.
No tears.
Just certainty.

I did not tell her how bad I believed things had become. I simply said I needed help with the kids and that my mom was exhausted.

She booked a plane ticket the next day.

And we continued waiting for the biopsy results.

Chapter 7 — Diagnosis

One evening, the oncologist came into the room and quietly told us the biopsy results.

Large B-Cell Lymphoma.

The bone marrow biopsy was still being analyzed, so they couldn't determine the stage yet. But one thing was already clear — the mass they had been calling a tumor was not a tumor at all. It was a cluster of massively enlarged lymph nodes.

That meant surgery was no longer an option.

All the surgical scenarios they had discussed were suddenly off the table. The only possible treatment now was chemotherapy.

The oncologist explained that this particular lymphoma often responds well to chemo. Depending on the stage, survival rates could reach as high as eighty-seven percent.

But my brain could barely process the words.
"Are you sure you can't operate?" I asked.

In that moment surgery almost sounded better.

The oncologist shook her head.

Even if they removed the lymph nodes, she explained, the disease was so aggressive that the cluster would likely return to the same size within forty-eight hours.

Chemotherapy was the only option.

That verdict hit even harder than the first phone call about the mango-sized mass.

The bone marrow results arrived the next day. They were clear. That meant Manuel was technically Stage II — bulky, but still Stage II.

It was good news… considering.

But all I could think about was chemotherapy.

I had been a holistic practitioner for seventeen years. Everything inside me resisted the idea. Every instinct, every belief system, every experience I had gathered over the years screamed no.

There had to be another way. Something better. Something less destructive.

And yet the reality in front of me was brutal.

Manuel could not hold down water. The enlarged lymph nodes were compressing his intestines and the duodenum, preventing liquids from moving through his digestive system. That was why everything he drank came back up.

And the cluster sat dangerously close to a major artery.

It was only a matter of time.
I interrogated that oncologist. But no matter how I tried to find another way there just was not any. I expressed my concern that

he is so weak now. How could his body handle chemotherapy right now? Would he even survive it?
And she was honest.

She said he might tolerate it, or he might not. But if we did nothing, he likely has days.

Days.

I had heard that before. In movies. In books. From clients repeating what doctors told them.
"You have four months."
"You have a few weeks."
It always made me angry.
Not because of the number — but because of what it did to people. It sounded like a sentence. Like a countdown.

Instead of saying:
You still have time.
You can fight.
Make changes.

But this time… I wasn't angry.
This time, it was real.
It wasn't months. It was days.
And I could see it with my own eyes. I knew — in our case — the doctor was right.

And that's when the real battle began.
Not in his body.
In my mind.

Everything I believed.
Everything I had taught.

Everything I had seen work.
Colliding with what was right in front of me.
Chemo… or no chemo.

The internal battle inside me was stronger than when we first heard the word cancer.

My mind flooded with everything I had seen over the years.

People who chose not to do chemotherapy and survived.
People who chose it and later said they wished they hadn't.

Stories. Opinions. Experiences.

Chris Wark and other survivors who had healed without it.

Even my own ego was loud.

How was I ever going to tell my clients that I signed the chemo papers?

I kept searching for another answer.

I called the oncologist in Mexico. I called integrative doctors I trusted. I asked every question I could think of.

But every conversation eventually led to the same reality.

"How are you going to give him juices and supplements," one of them asked, "if he can't even keep water down?"

That question stayed with me. Because it was true.

Without liquids moving through his system, nothing else could work.

At that point there were only two real options.

I could refuse chemotherapy… and watch him die.

Or I could see chemotherapy as another weapon — something that might buy us time.

Time to fight.

Time to support his body.

Time to do everything else.

That was the moment the decision became clear to me.

Not easy. Not peaceful.

Just clear.

But when the papers were finally placed in front of me, my body resisted.

Being the one who had to decide carried its own unbearable weight.
If the chemotherapy killed him that night, I would be the one who had signed the papers. I would be the one who had to tell the family that I made the choice that ended his life.

But if I refused it — if I let my beliefs or pride stand in the way and he died without even trying — I would carry that responsibility too.

How do you win in a situation like that?

It is one thing when the patient is making decisions for their own body. It is something entirely different when the responsibility falls on the spouse.

My hands started shaking.

I was hyperventilating.

The words on the page blurred through the tears filling my eyes. My chest felt tight, like a scream was stuck somewhere between my lungs and my throat.

I could barely see the paper.

But I signed.

The moment the pen left the page, the nurses moved with astonishing speed. They didn't walk — they ran. Within seconds the paperwork disappeared down the hallway and the preparation for chemotherapy began immediately.

There was no more time to think.

And just like that… it began.

Chapter 8 — The First Round

When the preparation for chemotherapy started, they sent me home.

They explained the possible reactions — allergic shock, seizures, other complications that could happen during the infusion. I was not allowed to stay. It was already past their Covid regulations and visiting limits.

The nurse promised she would call me when everything was over.

I kissed him on the forehead, told him to be strong, and left.

Home to a completely different battle.

They said the treatment would take about six hours.

I stayed awake and waited.

Every minute felt longer than the one before it.

Around one in the morning I called the hospital. My hands were shaking as I held the phone.

"He made it," the nurse said.

They had to revive him at one point, but he was alive.

I finally allowed myself to breathe.

The next morning I returned to the hospital.

When I walked into the room he looked almost the same as the day before — weak, pale, barely able to move.

Then the nurse casually announced that he was being discharged that day.

I stared at her.

"You're sending him home?"

He was vomiting constantly. He couldn't hold down water. They were about to remove his IV, and he could barely walk.

"And I'm supposed to take him home like this?"

They said yes.

The doctor explained that the first round of chemotherapy should begin shrinking the lymph nodes within a day or two. If that happened, the pressure on his digestive system might ease enough for liquids to pass through.

Hopefully.

A few hours later they wheeled him out of the hospital and into my car.

The drive home was only about twenty-five minutes, but we had to stop several times so he could vomit.

Somehow we made it home.

I helped him inside and took him straight to the bathroom. When I removed his clothes, I finally saw what had happened to his body.

Nothing had prepared me for that moment.

He weighed one hundred and fifteen pounds.

On a six-foot-tall man, that number barely seemed possible. His body looked like something I had only seen in historical photographs — prisoners from concentration camps, nothing but skin stretched over bone.

For a moment I simply stood there staring.

Then I helped him clean up and brought him to bed.

He was exhausted, but he kept smiling. He was happy to be home.

I told him to sleep.

Later that day I had him take tiny sips of water.

To my surprise, the water stayed down.

The next day his mother arrived. She came with one of his cousins and his wife. When they walked in, Manuel greeted them cheerfully — sitting upright, smiling, talking as if nothing unusual had happened.

They had no idea what he had just been through.

What *we* had just been through.

We told them only that he had spent three weeks in the hospital and received chemotherapy the day before. With clothes on, his weight loss wasn't as obvious. They talked for hours. Eventually his cousin and his wife left, but his mother stayed.

Little by little she began to understand the reality of the situation. Manuel still could not eat. The next day I made fresh juice — carrot, beet, and apple.

He sipped it slowly for almost an hour. And then something incredible happened. It stayed down. He remained on liquids for several more days while I slowly introduced small portions of vegan food. Tiny amounts at first. And they stayed down too. The chemotherapy had worked.

It hadn't cured anything yet, but it had done the one thing we desperately needed. It slowed the cancer down. Now we had time to fight. My confidence began to return.
And Manuel amazed me.

The very next day he was outside in the yard fixing something, cleaning, keeping himself busy. I stepped outside every few minutes reminding him to drink juice or water.

He played with the kids. His stamina and courage were almost impossible for me to understand.

I admired him more than ever.

Chemo had done the one thing we desperately needed.

It had bought us time.

And time meant we could fight.

Chapter 9 — The Fight

Death had stepped back, but it had not disappeared. The smell of it was gone, but the danger was still very real. The chemo had slowed the monster down, but it had not defeated it.

This was just the beginning.

Manuel weighed barely one hundred and fifteen pounds. The lymphoma had proven to be extremely aggressive, and chemotherapy itself carried its own risks. There was a lot working against us.

He was scheduled for six rounds of chemotherapy as an outpatient, followed by radiation treatments.

It was going to be a long battle.

From the beginning I knew we would approach this holistically. Conventional medicine and natural support did not have to be enemies. We didn't have to pick a side. We would use both.

And that's exactly what we did.

At that point I reminded Manuel of something we had already agreed on from the beginning.

"I will bring the weapons," I told him. "I will research, find what we need, and build the strategy."
"But you have to fight."

And he did.

Every day now had a structure. Healing was no longer an idea — it became a routine.

Once we realized that liquids were finally staying down, we started immediately. There was no reason to wait.

The protocol began that very day.

The first foundation was juice. Fresh vegetable juice became a daily ritual in our house. Manuel drank at least forty ounces every day. Carrot, beet, and apple were our main combination in the beginning — gentle enough for his stomach but powerful enough to nourish his body.

His diet became completely organic and almost entirely plant-based, with a strong focus on raw foods whenever he could tolerate them.

Twice a week he took a shot of wheatgrass juice. That one was rough. The taste alone could make your whole body protest, but we both knew how powerful it was. Sometimes healing is not pleasant, but it is necessary.

In the beginning we stuck mostly to liquid remedies because swallowing pills was still difficult for him. So many of the things I introduced came in drops, teas, or oils.

We learned about Essiac tea and its long history in cancer support *(details in Part 2)*. I started brewing it regularly, and he drank it three times a day.

Vitamin D with K2 came in liquid drops. Propolis drops were added as well, along with propolis cream that I applied directly over his abdomen. (*All details are explained in Part 2 of the book*) Black seed oil became another daily ritual.

I also began making my own yogurt using special bacterial cultures that I ordered. It technically wasn't vegan, but at that point supporting his gut mattered more than following perfect dietary rules. The homemade yogurt helped calm his stomach, especially after chemotherapy sessions.

Then there was the tea that became almost symbolic for us.

I ordered several herbs in bulk — sage, nettle, burdock root, dandelion, red clover, cat's claw, corn silk, chamomile, and peppermint. All of them carried anti-inflammatory and antioxidant properties.

One evening I mixed them together in proportions that simply felt right to me. I called it Healing Tea. Both of us drank it every day, and it quickly became something we looked forward to. The taste was warm and grounding.

Another remedy that became part of the routine was a simple asparagus preparation. I would cook the asparagus, blend it, store it in a glass jar in the refrigerator, and he would take four tablespoons twice a day.

And then there was the aloe juice.

Not the kind that sits on store shelves for months. This one came from a company that shipped it frozen overnight because it contained no preservatives at all. It was expensive, but it worked wonders for his digestive system and helped his gut recover after chemotherapy sessions.

Little by little, day by day, these things became our rhythm.

Healing became routine. And routines are powerful.

Time for his first outpatient treatment came quickly.

I took him to the clinic early in the morning for the long infusion. It was going to take most of the day. I packed juices and brought them with us, determined to keep supporting his body in every way I could.

Before we left, the oncologist gave me one clear instruction.

"If he develops a fever, take him to the ER immediately."

And he did.

The fever came the day after his second chemotherapy session. I took him to the emergency room. The testing seemed to take forever. Eventually they discovered that his white blood cell count had dropped to almost nothing. His immune system was practically gone.

They admitted him immediately and placed him in a sterile room. He spent another two weeks in the hospital.

During that time my life became a constant loop between home and the hospital, thirty minutes each way. I drove back and forth every day, sometimes twice a day. I brought him fresh juices and food each time.

Technically it wasn't allowed. The sterile room had strict rules about outside food. But I looked at the hospital trays and the microwaved meals they served and thought to myself that the food I was bringing was far cleaner than anything they were offering. So I brought it anyway.

He was receiving injections to stimulate his white blood cell production, and slowly it worked. His immune system began to recover, and eventually they released him.

When he came home we faced another moment.
His hair had started falling out everywhere. Not just on his head — from his entire body. Manuel had never been a particularly hairy man, but now hair was showing up on pillows, on clothes, in the shower.

So we shaved everything.

His head.
His arms.
His legs.

Even his eyebrows eventually fell out.

The kids watched with curiosity.

"Why, Mommy?" they asked.

We told them that Papi just wanted to see what he would look like bald. It was enough of an explanation for them, even though they clearly didn't love the new look.

While Manuel was in the hospital during that second round, something else happened at home.

Our five-year-old suddenly started wetting his bed.
It caught me off guard at first, but it was clear that even though we were trying to protect the kids from the full reality, they still felt the tension. Children always do.

I sat down with him and spoke gently.
"Yes, Papi isn't feeling well right now," I told him. "The doctors are fixing his stomach. It's not dangerous. He just needs some help." He listened quietly. And he trusted. The bedwetting stopped.

Through all of this, Manuel and I stayed focused on the fight.

He was taking at least ten different supplements at a time, rotating them every two weeks with another set so that we didn't overwhelm his system. He continued my cleansing protocols, drank fresh juice every day, and followed an organic plant-based diet.

We also incorporated the Hoxsey protocol — tonics and herbal supplements designed to support the body during cancer treatment.

Every three weeks he went through another round of chemotherapy.

After each round he took prednisone for five days, and once that cycle ended I took him to receive high-dose vitamin C IV therapy.

We started with 25 grams. Then 50. Eventually 100 grams, a four hour drip.

I even managed to obtain vitamin B17 from Mexico, and they added it to his vitamin C infusion bag.

Slowly, almost quietly, he began getting stronger.

And we kept dancing.

Tango had brought us together in the first place, and in the middle of all this it became a strange kind of anchor. Some evenings I was the one too exhausted to move, but he would still pull me up and we would dance in the living room.

For a few minutes everything else disappeared.

Chapter 10 — The Other Battles

While Manuel and I focused on treatments and the routines that were keeping him alive, life around us did not slow down.

In many ways it became even harder.

Cancer had entered our home, but it was not the only battle we were fighting.

Our financial situation quickly became a disaster.

Ironically, COVID ended up helping us in one small way. Because of the pandemic, mortgage forbearance programs were being offered. I applied for the hardship program and we were able to pause our mortgage payments for twelve months.

Without that, I honestly don't know what we would have done.

Before Manuel went into the hospital we had maybe ten thousand dollars in savings. We had always lived reasonably well. With his business and my practice we were doing fine — not rich, but comfortably middle class. That ended quickly.

The savings disappeared fast. I still had some clients, but my energy simply wasn't there anymore. Between hospital visits, treatments, the kids, and trying to hold everything together, work became almost impossible.

Money was draining quickly.

The hospital treatments were mostly covered by insurance, but all the natural treatments I was adding — supplements, herbs, vitamin C infusions, special foods — cost thousands.

A couple of Manuel's friends helped us a few times, which was a blessing. But mostly we were on our own. And I decided not to tell Manuel how bad things were financially.

He had enough to carry already. The last thing he needed was to carry that burden too. So I carried it myself. To this day I don't fully understand how we managed it. Somehow we did.

With God's help, things kept working out just enough to keep moving forward. But the loans and the debt from that time are still with us. Money was not the only storm happening in our home.

My oldest son was going through his own collapse. He failed every class that third quarter. Even gym. He started spending time with the wrong friends and finished his freshman year in complete disaster. The boy who had spent eleven years playing violin, practicing, performing, building friendships through music, suddenly quit everything.
School stopped mattering. Home stopped mattering. He became defiant. It was painful to watch.

I knew some of it came from fear and stress. He had already lost his biological father when he was younger, and now he was watching his stepfather fight the disease that to most people sounds like a verdict.

But in that moment I desperately needed him to rise up and be strong for the family — for his younger brothers, for me. Instead, he began slipping away.

I eventually had to pull him out of school and transfer him to homeschooling. I thought it might protect him from bad influences and help him reset. I had no idea that he had already found ways around my control.

He started sneaking out of the house at night, crawling out of his bedroom window and meeting up with a friend who was getting him into trouble. The police knocking on our door became part of our reality. He was arrested once and released a few hours later with probation. Three weeks later — on his sixteenth birthday — it happened again. Again he was released. Again probation.

None of the charges were anything truly serious, but at the time it felt like the end of the world for me. I knew I had loosened the leash too much.

I had allowed certain things simply because I did not have the energy left to fight every battle. Between Manuel's illness, the treatments, the financial stress, and the younger kids, I was exhausted. I trusted that the foundation I had given him growing up would be strong enough to hold.

But his own fear and stress had their own rules. He was terrified too. He just expressed it in the only way a teenager sometimes knows how — rebellion.

We talked. We spent time together. I tried to show him the strength Manuel was demonstrating every day.
Sometimes it worked. Sometimes it didn't.

And through all of it, I carried that weight too.
Another layer of stress.
Another layer of grief.
Another layer of overwhelm.

Chapter 11 — The Angel in the Sky

After Manuel came home from his second hospital stay, we decided to take the kids to the beach. We all needed air. Space. Something that felt normal again.

I was driving. The boys were laughing in the back seat, happy just to be out of the house. The sky was bright and clear, one of those perfect Florida days.

But my mind was somewhere else.

Inside my head I kept repeating the same thought over and over like a prayer.

I need to know that he is going to be okay.
I need a sign that he is going to live.

At that exact moment I was making a right turn onto the bridge going to the key. And suddenly my jaw dropped.

Right in front of me in the sky, the clouds had formed a huge white angel.

The clouds were very thin, almost transparent, and the sun sat perfectly where the head would be. It was so clear that for a moment I wondered if I was imagining it.

But I wasn't.

I even managed to take a picture.

I just smiled. Then I turned to Manuel and said quietly, "You're going to be just fine."

He saw it. He felt it. He knew it.

Everything we had gone through, everything we were learning, everything Manuel was doing for his health began leading him closer to God.

He was going to church regularly. A Spanish-speaking church felt natural for him. He noticed that on the days he went, he felt better — calmer, stronger, more hopeful.

His faith began to grow. And with it, his strength.

We continued the cycle we had created.

Chemotherapy.
Prednisone.
Cleansing.
Vitamin C IV infusions.
Supplements.
Prayer.
Church.
Affirmations.

And then we repeated it again.

The additional support we were giving his body made a tremendous difference. He did not experience the severe side effects that many people associate with chemotherapy.

He wasn't vomiting.

He didn't feel constant nausea.
He had no digestive pain.

Instead, he stayed active.

He was always doing something — building something, fixing something around the house, playing soccer with the kids in the yard.

I could see the immediate effect of the vitamin C infusions. He would go in looking pale, almost yellowish, with dark circles under his eyes. Five hours later he would come out with clear eyes and color back in his face.

It was impressive to watch.

One side effect he did experience was nerve damage in the tips of his fingers. He lost some feeling there, which meant that sometimes he would accidentally hurt himself while working with tools — a hammer here, a sharp edge there.

But even that didn't slow him down much.
He kept moving.

He kept working.

He kept living.

Chapter 12 — The Final Shot

Four months later, after all the rounds of chemotherapy were completed, his blood work looked good. The scans looked good too. For the first time in a long while, there was a sense of relief.

But the doctors were not finished.

They strongly recommended radiation.

Twenty-five rounds directed at his abdomen. They called it a final shot to the area — a way to fully deactivate the cluster of lymph nodes where the lymphoma had grown.

I thought about it for a long time.

There was a lot of resistance inside me.

And honestly, even today I am still not completely convinced it was the right decision.

The radiologist explained that radiation damage continues for years. The tissue keeps scarring, sometimes for up to ten years. Some patients later develop colon blockages from that scarring.

Listening to that explanation was terrifying.

It sounded harsh. Permanent. Unnecessary.

But then there was the other side of the argument.

What if we didn't do it?

The oncologists warned that if the lymphoma returned, the same chemotherapy would no longer work. The next option would likely be a bone marrow transplant — a procedure that costs hundreds of thousands of dollars and carries its own enormous risks.

The message between the lines was clear. If it comes back, you may not have another chance.

Suddenly I found myself in the same mental spiral I had faced when deciding about chemotherapy. Only this time it was even harder.

Manuel was no longer helpless in a hospital bed. He was walking, working, functioning again. He was fully capable of making his own decision. But he still looked to me for guidance. And somehow, once again, it felt like the final call was mine.

For weeks radiation became the only topic in our house.

I interrogated the oncologist. I questioned the radiologist. I scheduled consultations with integrative doctors we trusted. I spoke with the oncologist in Mexico we had been working with throughout the process.

The oncologist and radiologist spoke mostly from fear — explaining the risks of recurrence and the limitations if the cancer returned.

The integrative doctors were more neutral. They could discuss possibilities and support the conversation, but none of them were willing to take responsibility for the decision.

And honestly, how could they?

No one was going to sign those papers except us.

The responsibility had to stay where it belonged.

With him. With us. We talked about it for weeks.

We weighed every possibility.

If he agreed to radiation, we knew there would be irreversible damage. His body had already been through chemotherapy. Radiation would add another layer of harm, another risk for the future. Secondary cancers are a known possibility after heavy radiation exposure.

But if he refused it — and the lymphoma returned stronger — we would have to live with that question forever.

What if the radiation could have prevented it?

We drove ourselves nearly insane going back and forth.
In the end, Manuel made the decision.

He agreed to the radiation.

Radiation treatments began soon after the decision was made.

Twenty-five sessions.

Five days a week. Monday through Friday. For five weeks.

Compared to chemotherapy, each individual treatment was short. The actual radiation itself took only about fifteen minutes. But the routine around it became part of our daily life.

Every morning I drove him to the clinic.

We checked in, waited our turn, and then he went in alone while I sat in the waiting room. The machine would do its work, and shortly after he would come back out and we would drive home again.

At first it didn't seem too bad.

But radiation works differently than chemotherapy. The effect builds day after day, and by the second or third week the cumulative toll became obvious.

He definitely felt weaker. Much weaker than he had during most of the chemotherapy.

Every afternoon when we came home, I had the same routine waiting for him. I prepared a detox bath.

I mixed baking soda, Dead Sea salt, and Epsom salt — a cup of each — into warm water. Our bathtub was small and his six-foot body didn't fit perfectly, but I made sure his torso stayed fully submerged while his legs rested outside.

He soaked there for twenty minutes.

The baths helped draw out toxins, relax his body, and give him at least some relief from the constant buildup of treatment.

At the same time, we continued everything else we had already built into our routine.

Fresh juices every day. Supplements. Herbal support.

And once a week he went in for a high-dose vitamin C IV infusion.

The goal was always the same: support his body as much as possible while the treatments did their work.

We counted the sessions one by one.

Twenty-five treatments.
Twenty-four.
Twenty-three.

Every day brought us one step closer to the end.
And finally, the last session arrived.

When it was finished, we walked out of the clinic quietly. There was no celebration, no dramatic moment.

Just a quiet understanding between us that the most intense phase of the battle was finally behind us.

The treatments were over.

Chapter 13 — Chemo Brain

One of the hardest parts of the recovery was not physical.

Physically, Manuel was slowly getting stronger. His faith was growing. His body was stabilizing after everything it had been through.

But something else had changed. His mind.

It was difficult to watch what chemotherapy had done to his brain function.

For almost a full year I could not let him drive. I drove everywhere — to appointments, treatments, errands. I scheduled everything. I handled every detail of daily life.

On the surface he seemed mostly fine. But when you paid attention, something was clearly wrong. If someone asked him for his birth date, he might give them his zip code. If they asked for his phone number, random numbers would come out.

I am not exaggerating.

He could speak, but information was constantly getting mixed up. Sometimes he couldn't even spell his own name out loud.

English, which had been perfectly manageable for him before, almost disappeared. He simply couldn't find the words. But when he spoke Spanish with his family, he could talk for hours.

Watching that was confusing and frightening at the same time. Slowly, after chemotherapy ended, the words started coming back.

I waited patiently.

Still, about a year later he was not fully himself yet. The oncologist and I even discussed whether we should scan his brain to make sure nothing else was happening. In the end I decided not to.

There were no other signs pointing to cancer in his head, and the last thing I wanted was to expose him to more radiation unnecessarily. So we waited.

Little by little, things began improving.

Eventually he started driving again. He began thinking about what kind of work he should do going forward. We suspected that the lymphoma may have been related to the chemicals he had been exposed to for years working in construction.

So he tried exploring other options. He picked up small jobs here and there. Nothing close to the income we had before, but it was a start and it felt like progress.

At one point he even tried window tinting for cars. He liked it, but it was a completely new business to build.

Then another reality became clear. The nerve damage in his fingertips — another side effect from chemotherapy — made delicate work extremely difficult. Without full sensation in his fingers, it took him far too long to complete even simple tasks.

So that idea had to be set aside as well. But the body was still healing.

Slowly, almost quietly, feeling started returning to his fingertips — one finger at a time. It was a small sign, but it meant something important. His nerves were rebuilding. His body was rebuilding. And with every small improvement, hope grew stronger.

The Dream

Not long after the radiation treatments ended, something happened that stayed with both of us.

One night Manuel suddenly sat up in bed in the middle of the night. His breathing was heavy and his whole body was sweating. The movement woke me up.

He had just had a nightmare.

In the dream a huge monster attacked him — an octopus with massive tentacles. The tentacles wrapped around his body, and the suction cups were attached exactly to his abdomen, right where the "tumor" had been.

It was a spiritual battle.

He struggled to break free while the creature held onto him. In the dream he began praying, and then he shouted at it:

"I am not afraid of you!"

And just like that, the monster disappeared into thin air.

When he told me what had happened, I listened quietly.

Then I said something that surprised even me.

“Oh good,” I told him calmly. “I’ve been waiting for this dream. It’s all gone now. No more cancer.”

And I fell back asleep.

In the morning we talked about it again.

What was that?

I have always been a very intuitive person, and over the years I’ve experienced moments where messages seemed to arrive in ways that are difficult to explain logically.

This felt like one of those moments.

We both knew what the dream meant.

He had won.

The war was over.

Life slowly began returning to something that resembled normal. We continued the routines that had helped him heal — the diet, the supplements, the care — but the intensity was no longer the same.

The battle had been fought.

The “monster" had disappeared.

Chapter 14 — Living Through the Battle

Things were still rough.

Manuel was alive, but he was not the same man he had been before the illness. Stress was still high, and yet somehow, through all of it, we were still happy.

Looking back at the pictures from that time makes me wonder how we did it. There we are — smiling, dancing, going to the beach, playing with the kids.

How did we find the energy?
How did we keep going?

More than anything, I remember how impressed I was with the man I had chosen. I was proud of him.

How could someone go through something like that and still stay so positive?

And how could I — a person who had never been known for unlimited patience — stay so focused and determined?

When I look back, the physical contrast is shocking.

He was not the man I had met.

The man I met was big, tall, with olive skin. I used to jokingly call him "Sexicano." We met through tango, and tango has a way of building passion quickly.

Our relationship was built on movement, energy, and intensity.

Now he looked like a completely different person.

He was bald, pale, incredibly thin — almost skeletal. At one point he weighed almost the same as me, and I am only five foot three. His mind was slower, his body fragile.

But he was still smiling. And his passion for life had actually grown stronger. Even his passion for me had not changed.

Maybe that was what carried us through. We kept living. We danced in the living room. We went to the beach. We played with the kids. Was everything cheerful and easy?

Of course not.

Finances were screaming. Loans were piling up.
Some of his teeth had begun falling out from the treatments. Not all of them, but enough that he needed partials. There was a period of time when he was waiting for them, and I remember feeling embarrassed sometimes when people looked at him.

He looked so thin. So old.

He had gone from always looking younger than his age to looking like he was eighty. Sometimes when we walked the kids to school, I felt like people staring.

He looked more like a grandfather than a father. That part was emotionally difficult. But whenever those thoughts appeared, I grounded myself in something else.

I remembered who he was just a few months earlier. I remembered how we met. I remembered the way we danced. And I reminded myself that healing takes time.

Maybe he would never be exactly the same again. But I believed he could come close. And in many ways, he surprised me.

We would go on family bike rides in the evenings. We had one of those baby carts attached to the back of the bike for our youngest. The kid was not exactly light anymore — almost three years old and pretty chunky.

But Manuel would pull him. I couldn't even do it. It was too heavy for me. But he did it. Even while still going through treatment. Every evening we rode around the neighborhood and the kids loved it. On Sundays we rode our bikes to the organic farm stand that we were lucky enough to have nearby. It was about a fifteen-minute ride. On the way back we would load the baby cart with bags of vegetables — bags and a kid — and Manuel still pulled it all the way home.

He refused to let me carry the heavy things. How could anyone not be in love with that?

But darkness did come sometimes.

I would be lying if I said it didn't.

There were moments when I felt sorry for myself. Moments when I asked why life had turned this way.

Why did we have to go through something like this?

But those thoughts never stayed for long.

I knew too well that falling into a victim mentality would only dig a deeper hole for all of us.

So every time those thoughts appeared, I would bring myself back to the same questions:

Who were we before this?

Who could we still become?

And what needed to be done today?

That mindset carried us forward.

Sometimes life places unbearable responsibility in our hands.

And only later do we realize that being trusted with that responsibility was also a form of privilege.

Chapter 15 — Another Scare

According to the oncologist, the cancer would be considered cured if it stayed away for three years. After that, he said he would only need to see Manuel once a year for basic blood work. Even the scans would no longer be necessary.

That three-year mark became an invisible finish line in our minds.

It was November 2023 — two years since all treatments had finished, and almost three years since the nightmare had started. Manuel went in for what was supposed to be his last six-month scan before switching to yearly follow-ups.

We were excited. Then the scan came back with terrifying news.

A lesion had appeared on his lung.

They couldn't say exactly what it was, but they explained that when this particular lymphoma returns, it often shows up in the lungs. They recommended a biopsy as soon as possible.

Everything stopped. Panic. Frustration. Disbelief.

After everything we had already gone through, this felt like being pushed back to the beginning again.
I called a close friend of mine whose father had just passed away from colon cancer. We talked. We cried for a moment.

But then something shifted.

I remembered the dream. The monster disappearing.

I remembered the angel in the sky from years earlier.

And despite the terrifying language doctors tend to use — language that often multiplies fear — something inside me stayed calm.

"No," I said. "I don't think it's cancer."

It could be anything. Manuel had been sick shortly before the scan. It could have been inflammation, infection, even leftover effects from COVID.

Other than that small spot on the scan, he felt completely fine.

So I made a decision.

"Let's do the biopsy," I said. "But schedule it one month from now."

The risks were real. A lung biopsy can collapse the lung. But I wasn't afraid of waiting a few weeks. The biopsy was scheduled for mid-December.

In the meantime, I put Manuel back on a protocol.
One quart of carrot juice every day. Carrot juice has remarkable cleansing and restorative properties.

I also started researching something I had recently heard about — nicotine's possible interaction with certain viral mechanisms. After listening to a lecture by Dr. Ardis and digging deeper into the research myself, the idea made more and more sense.

So for thirty days Manuel followed a simple routine:

Four cups of carrot juice daily.
Back to a strict vegan diet.
And a 7 mg nicotine patch each day.

Thirty days passed.

He went in for the biopsy.

Then we waited. And waited.

It was taking far longer than expected.

Christmas Eve arrived.

I was walking into Whole Foods to grab a few last-minute things when my phone rang. It was a random number. Normally I would ignore it — most unknown calls are scams — but something made me answer.

It was Sarah, the oncologist's nurse practitioner.

My heart dropped.
She immediately said, "I'm not at the office — we're closed for the holidays — but I checked the emails and saw Manuel's results. I had to call you. It's Christmas and you deserve to know."

I leaned against a display of small Christmas trees outside the store while people walked past me staring.

"The biopsy is back," she said.

"It is NOT cancer."

She continued explaining that the reason it had taken so long was because the pathologists were trying to understand what the tissue actually was. They had tested it for tuberculosis and several other possibilities.

In the end, all they could say was that it was dead tissue.

Dead tissue.

I remember thinking: Who cares what it was?

Whatever it had been — it was dead.

We had killed it.

I planned to tell Manuel when I got home, but I couldn't wait. I called him immediately.

I tried to speak quickly so I wouldn't scare him.

"Sarah just called me," I said. "It's not cancer. I'll explain everything when I get home."

Even that sentence scared him at first.

But when he understood what I meant, he cried.

Not from fear.

From relief.

It was the best Christmas gift we could have received.

Experiences like this change your understanding of what a "gift" really is.

Jewelry, gadgets, holiday presents — they suddenly feel meaningless compared to something as simple as a doctor saying, "Your biopsy is clear."

The gift is life.

Nothing else really comes close.

And living through something like this changes the way you see your role in the story.

Technically, this was Manuel's illness.

He was the patient.

But somehow the entire journey had become mine too.

Whenever I talk about those years, I never say he did this or he went through that.

I always say we.
We did this.
We went there.
We fought this.

Was I just a caregiver?

A practitioner making decisions?

Or had walking through the battle beside him made me a patient in my own way as well?

Chapter 16 — When the War Ends

As strong as I stayed through all of it, at some point the energy shifted.

For years I had simply kept moving. Decisions had to be made. Treatments had to be organized. The house had to run. The kids had to be taken care of. There was no time to fall apart.

But eventually the body keeps its own record of what the mind refuses to process.

And mine started speaking.

The first signal was my back.

The pain appeared suddenly, deep in my lower back. Sitting became impossible. The only positions that gave relief were standing or lying flat. Walking was manageable, but every day became a strange rotation between those two positions.

I tried everything — acupuncture, massage, chiropractors.
At first nothing helped.

One chiropractor eventually managed to calm the pain, but not before several scans and tests. At one point I was convinced something serious was wrong with me. My abdomen felt tight and swollen. Everything hurt.

CT scans and ultrasounds showed nothing.
Finally an MRI revealed the answer.

Two herniated discs.

After two months of intense pain I slowly improved. But exactly one year later the pain returned again. That episode lasted about a month before stabilizing, and since then I have never felt fully the same. One wrong movement can bring the pain back.

Sleep has become another battle. Most nights I fall asleep normally, but around four in the morning the pain wakes me up. My back begins pulling and aching and suddenly rest becomes impossible. I turn from side to side, exhausted but unable to sleep.

At first I thought this was purely physical. But something else had begun shifting as well. My emotions. I became more irritated.

The same man I had spent years admiring — the man I had watched fight cancer with such strength — suddenly began irritating me.

His mental slowness, which I had patiently accepted during recovery, now frustrated me. He was functioning again. He worked, brought income, helped with the kids.
And yet everything seemed to annoy me. Sometimes he would say quietly, "It feels like anything I say irritates you."

And I would answer honestly.

"It does."

But I also knew something else.

"It's probably not you. It's probably me."

Was it hormones? Perimenopause? Exhaustion?

I started observing myself the way I observe my clients. Looking for patterns. And one word kept appearing.

Responsibility.

That word sat heavy in my body. I was managing everything.

Appointments.
Finances.
Groceries.
School decisions.
Family schedules.

Everything passed through me.

And slowly I began seeing a strange parallel.
In autoimmune disease the immune system becomes overwhelmed. It works harder and harder until it begins attacking the body itself.

I started wondering if there was something similar happening emotionally. Some kind of autoimmune emotional management disease.

For years I had been managing everyone and everything. Over time that management had turned into micromanagement.
And now I was attacking everyone around me for it.

Cancer had been gone for years. Five years officially.
But those five years felt like an entire lifetime.

When I finally stopped long enough to look back, I realized something important.

Cancer had not been the only storm during those years. It had simply been the biggest one.

Right after chemotherapy and radiation ended we discovered a leak in our kitchen. The floor literally began lifting. When the cabinets were removed we discovered massive mold contamination. Our insurance company told us to leave the house immediately.

So we did.
We moved between Airbnbs while remediation dragged on for months. Eventually we fired the company handling it, and Manuel — who had just finished chemotherapy and radiation — rebuilt the house himself with help from friends.

Six months after moving back in, I decided I wanted out of that house entirely. We sold it and bought another one.

Around the same time our middle son broke his femur in a park accident. There were ambulance rides, hospital transfers, two surgeries, and months in a wheelchair. Manuel carried him everywhere — to the bathroom, the bathtub, the car.

Then there was my oldest son.

A boy who had once been deeply dedicated to violin and youth orchestra began unraveling. Failed classes, new friends, arrests, court dates, probation. Nothing extremely serious — but enough to make a mother feel like everything was collapsing.

When Manuel became sick, my son's only reaction had been one sentence:

"Am I going to lose another dad?"

That night I prayed harder than I ever had before. But to my son I said something with certainty.

"No. This one will live."

And he did. But the boy shut down emotionally in ways I still don't fully understand.

Meanwhile our finances were collapsing.

Manuel's business had lost most of its clients during his illness. My own practice was barely running because I had no energy left to give.

Two years after Manuel's diagnosis, my father was diagnosed with bladder cancer. Two years later he was gone.

And somewhere in the middle of everything, the investment property we had planned to flip began sliding into foreclosure.

Looking back now, I see what I couldn't see then.
It wasn't just cancer. It was everything.
Storm after storm after storm.

There was simply no space between them to stop and process any of it. I just kept pushing forward like a train without brakes.
Until my body finally forced me to stop.

When Manuel had to travel to Mexico for three weeks.

People kept asking me the same question:

"How are you managing everything without him?"

At first I answered casually.

Then suddenly it hit me.

Nothing had changed. My life was exactly the same.

The house still ran the same way. The kids still came to me for everything. All the decisions were still mine. The only difference was that no one was sleeping next to me at night.

That realization landed heavily.

What was the point of this marriage if I was still dragging everything alone?

During Manuel's illness I had taken control of everything because someone had to. He learned to follow instructions. I learned to give them. At the time it saved his life. Years later it was exhausting mine.

When he came home from Mexico I was happy to see him, but resentment that had been quietly growing for years suddenly surfaced.

Instead of expressing it calmly, I attacked.

"You live only for yourself."

"You bring a paycheck but don't even ask if the bills are paid."

"Why is everything still on me?"

At one point I even said something harsh.

"If it wasn't for the kids, we probably wouldn't even be together."

His response was simple.

"Yeah, probably."

And strangely, it didn't hurt.

Because by that point I already knew something uncomfortable.

I had become difficult to live with. Sharp. Angry. Exhausted.
But the real question wasn't whether I had changed. The real question was why.

The truth was that both of us were still living inside the roles we learned during the war. I kept running, carrying everything on my back. And he walked beside me enjoying the sunshine, wondering why the donkey was unhappy.

It sounds funny now. But at the time it wasn't. Eventually we began adjusting. He asked me to give him specific responsibilities. So I did. Three things he now handles every day.
The kids are learning something too. For years everything was "Mama, mama, mama." Now when they come to me first, I simply say:

"Go ask Papi."

Little by little the balance is shifting.
Because surviving the war was only the first step.
Learning how to live after it is another battle entirely.

Chapter 17 — What the War Taught Me

When people hear our story, they usually focus on the cancer.

The diagnosis.
The hospital.
The chemotherapy.

But cancer was only the most visible part of the war. The real battle was something deeper. It was the moment when life suddenly placed responsibility in our hands and asked a very simple question:

What are you going to do now?

There is a moment in every crisis when panic is possible, when fear can take over and paralyze everything. But fear is not a strategy.

Very early in Manuel's illness I realized something important: we did not have the luxury of fear. Fear drains energy, and energy was the one thing we could not afford to lose.
So we focused on action.
Every day there were decisions to make.
Doctors to question.
Treatments to research.
Food to prepare.
Protocols to build.

Some of those decisions were terrifying. Signing the chemotherapy papers was one of them. Even now, years later, I can still feel the weight of that moment. But once the decision was made, the next step was simple.

Move forward. That became our rule.

We didn't waste time asking why this had happened to us. We didn't spend energy imagining worst-case scenarios. We focused on what could be done today.

Today we drink the juice.
Today we take the supplements.
Today we pray.
Today we rest.
Today we fight.

One step at a time.

Another thing the war taught me is that healing is rarely about choosing one side. People love simple answers. They want to believe that either conventional medicine or natural medicine holds the truth. But life is rarely that simple.

In our case, chemotherapy bought us time. Without it, Manuel likely would not have survived long enough for anything else to work. At the same time, nutrition, cleansing, supplements, and emotional strength supported his body in ways medicine alone could not.

It was never a battle between two systems. It was a partnership. We used every tool available.

Another lesson became clear again and again: the patient's will matters more than anything else. I had seen it before in my work with clients. People who recover from serious illness almost always share one common trait.

They decide to live.
Not hope.
Not wish.
Decide.

Manuel never allowed himself to fall into a victim mentality. Even at his weakest moments he kept moving — fixing things around the house, playing with the kids, dancing with me in the living room. Some people might say that attitude was simply his personality.

Maybe.

But I believe it was also a choice. And that choice mattered.

For me personally, the war also revealed something else. Responsibility can feel unbearable when it is suddenly placed on your shoulders. During Manuel's illness I often felt overwhelmed by the number of decisions I had to make.

Looking back now, I understand something I could not see at the time. Being trusted with that responsibility was also a form of privilege.

Life had placed someone I loved in my care and asked me to step forward. Not everyone receives that kind of trust.

The experience also reminded me of something fundamental about the body.

The body is not our enemy.

It is an intelligent system constantly trying to protect and adapt. When we support it properly — through nourishment, detoxification, rest, emotional stability, and faith — it has an extraordinary ability to recover.

That recovery is rarely instant.

But it is real.

Over the years many people have asked me the same question:

What exactly did you do?
What did Manuel eat?
What supplements did he take?
What treatments helped the most?

The truth is there was no single miracle solution.

What helped was a system.

A strategy.

A protocol built from many small decisions repeated every single day. And that is what I want to share next.

Because while every illness and every person is different, the principles behind that protocol can help many people support their bodies during serious illness.

The war taught us how to fight.

What comes next is the map we followed.

Part II

The Strategy

Up to this point, you have read our story.
A very personal story — one family walking through the shock of diagnosis, the chaos of treatment, and the slow climb back toward life.
When people hear our story, they often ask the same question.

What exactly did you do?

What did Manuel eat?
What supplements did he take?
What treatments helped him recover?
What made the difference?

The truth is that there was never a single miracle solution.

There was no one pill, no one therapy, no one moment that suddenly changed everything.

What helped was a system.

A strategy built from many small decisions repeated every single day.

Some of those decisions came from my professional background as a holistic practitioner. Others came from research, conversations with doctors, books, intuition, and sometimes simple observation of how the body responds when it is supported instead of burdened.

We used conventional medicine when it was necessary.
We used natural approaches wherever we could.
We paid attention to food, detoxification, supplements, mindset, faith, and daily discipline.

Nothing worked alone.

Everything worked together.

During the months of treatment our lives became structured around one simple goal:

Create the best possible conditions for the body to recover.

Every meal mattered.
Every supplement had a purpose.
Every habit either helped or hindered healing.

Over time those daily choices became a protocol.

Not a rigid formula that works for every person in every situation, but a framework — a way of thinking about health, healing, and the body's remarkable ability to regenerate when given the right environment.

What follows in the next chapters is not a universal prescription.

It is the strategy we used.

The principles that guided our decisions.
The tools that supported Manuel's recovery.
The practices that helped his body endure aggressive medical treatment while still rebuilding strength.

Every person's journey is different. Every illness has its own complexity.

But the body's basic needs remain the same:

Remove unnecessary burdens.
Provide clean nourishment.
Support detoxification.
Strengthen the immune system.
Protect the mind and spirit.

Healing begins when the body is finally given the conditions it needs to do what it was designed to do.

The following chapters walk through the most important parts of that strategy — beginning with the foundation of all healing:

Nutrition.

Chapter 18 — Foundation of Healing

By the time Manuel came home from the hospital, nutrition had already become one of the central parts of our strategy.

In our house we were already eating organically and had a strong awareness of chemical exposure. Since that very first phone call, he had been on a strict healing diet. Fresh foods, cleansing cycles, juicing, and plant-based meals were not new to him. They had been part of our life for years.

Yet during his hospital stay a very different approach was presented. Because of his dramatic weight loss, a hospital dietitian was sent to speak with him. She brought a printed list of foods he should begin eating immediately in order to regain weight.

The focus was simple:

Calories.

The list included dairy products, burgers, fried foods, ice cream, and other high-calorie options intended to help him gain weight as quickly as possible.

I remember looking at that list in complete disbelief.

At that moment Manuel's body was in the middle of a severe biological crisis. His digestive system was barely functioning, he could hardly keep liquids down, and his organs were under enormous stress. And yet the solution offered was to load the body with the heaviest foods possible.

It raised a question that stayed with me long after that conversation. Does anyone stop to ask why the body loses so much weight during a crisis?

The body is intelligent. When survival is at stake, it often sheds unnecessary burden. Digestion is one of the most energy-intensive processes in the body. Heavy foods demand enormous metabolic effort.

Weight loss during illness may not simply be failure. In many cases it may be the body's attempt to redirect energy toward survival. Yet the system often focuses almost entirely on restoring weight as quickly as possible, without considering the metabolic cost of the foods used to do it.

For us, the question was not how quickly Manuel could gain weight. The question was how we could support the body's healing mechanisms while keeping digestion as light and efficient as possible.

That meant nutrition could not simply be about calories. It had to be about biology.

True Healing Nutrition

True healing nutrition is not complicated. It is disciplined simplicity.

The human body is not designed to interpret dozens of ingredients at once. Each food carries its own chemical, enzymatic, and energetic signature. When too many foods are introduced simultaneously — even if they are individually healthy — the digestive system becomes overwhelmed.

Efficiency drops, and the organs responsible for filtration and elimination must compensate.

This is why complex meals often lead to fatigue, heaviness, bloating, and long-term metabolic strain. Healing nutrition moves in the opposite direction. It simplifies.

The Body Thrives on Clarity

Simple meals allow the stomach to secrete the appropriate acids, the pancreas to release the correct enzymes, and the intestines to absorb nutrients efficiently.

Complexity creates competition inside the digestive system.

Simplicity creates nourishment.

When digestion becomes easier, the body can redirect energy toward repair, immune function, and detoxification rather than spending it entirely on processing food.

Ingredient Integrity

The body recognizes food — not chemistry.

Anything artificial that enters the body must be neutralized, transformed, or eliminated. Artificial colors, preservatives, pesticides, solvents, medications, smoke, alcohol, and environmental toxins all pass through the bloodstream and must ultimately be filtered — primarily by the liver.

The liver's role is not only to process nutrients but to protect the blood from substances that do not belong in it.

Over time, chemical exposures accumulate and begin to burden the body's natural filtration systems.
This is why ingredient quality matters.
Whenever possible, foods should be:

- Organic
- Whole
- Minimally processed
- Fresh
- Free of chemical additives

This is not a lifestyle trend.
It is a physiological necessity when the body is attempting to heal.

Living vs. Depleted Nutrition

Fresh plant foods carry biological vitality.

Vegetables, fruits, greens, sprouts, and whole plant foods contain enzymes, structured water, antioxidants, and micronutrients that participate directly in cellular repair.

Highly processed foods may still contain calories, but their biological intelligence has largely been stripped away. Refining, preserving, and excessive heating reduce enzyme activity and nutritional integrity.

These foods require digestive effort while contributing very little to regeneration. Healing occurs most efficiently when the majority of the diet consists of fresh, living foods.

A plant-based diet in this context is not a moral position. It is a biological one.

Animal protein is dense, slow to digest, and metabolically demanding. During intensive healing phases, reducing that digestive burden allows the body to redirect energy toward detoxification and repair.

The Protein Myth

Fear of protein deficiency is largely cultural rather than physiological.

All plants contain amino acids. Many plant foods — especially leafy greens, legumes, quinoa, buckwheat, seeds, and nuts — provide protein in highly usable forms.

Unlike animal protein, which must be extensively broken down before assimilation, plant proteins are absorbed with less metabolic strain and fewer toxic byproducts.
True strength is not built through overload.
It is built through efficient nourishment.

Juicing as Cellular Nutrition

Juicing is not a trend.

It is therapeutic nutrition.

Fresh juices deliver minerals, vitamins, enzymes, and phytochemicals in a form that is rapidly absorbed. Because the fiber is removed, the digestive system does not have to break down plant structure before nutrients enter the bloodstream.

This is especially valuable during illness, when digestion may already be compromised.

Juices are best consumed on an empty stomach.
Vegetable juices form the foundation, with fruit used sparingly for balance and palatability.

Common combinations we used included:

- carrot juice
- carrot and celery
- carrot, beet, green apple, and lemon
- carrot, cucumber, and lemon
- carrot with leafy greens such as kale

Small amounts of ginger and turmeric root were often added for their anti-inflammatory and antimicrobial properties.

However, both are very potent. Ginger can become extremely spicy when juiced, and turmeric can easily overpower the flavor if used in excess.

Balance matters.

Intelligent Hydration

Hydration should begin early in the day.

A glass of room-temperature water upon waking prepares the digestive system and supports circulation. Many people benefit from adding fresh lemon juice, apple cider vinegar, or a small pinch of mineral-rich salt to help restore electrolyte balance.

Modern filtration removes harmful substances from water but often strips away beneficial minerals as well.

Adding a small amount of natural mineral salt can help restore this balance. More water is not always better.

Excessive intake of demineralized water can dilute electrolytes and reduce cellular hydration.

Balance matters.

Inflammation or Nourishment

Every meal produces a response inside the body.

Some foods calm tissues, improve circulation, and reduce inflammation. Others create irritation, congestion, and metabolic stress.

Foods that commonly increase inflammatory load include:

- refined sugar
- ultra-processed foods
- excessive animal fats
- processed meats
- artificial additives and preservatives
- heavily fried foods
- refined vegetable oils

On the other hand, many foods actively support anti-inflammatory processes:

- fresh vegetables and leafy greens
- root vegetables such as carrots, beets, sweet potatoes, and turnips
- herbs and spices like ginger, turmeric, cumin, garlic, and cinnamon

- berries and deeply colored fruits
- raw nuts and seeds
- fresh herbs

These foods contain antioxidants and phytonutrients that help calm inflammatory pathways and support cellular repair.
A healing diet is defined not only by nutrients, but also by how the body feels after eating. When food consistently leaves the body clearer, lighter, and more stable, healing is taking place.

Food as Biological Information

Food is more than fuel.

Every meal communicates with the immune system, hormones, the nervous system, and metabolism. It influences inflammation, blood sugar regulation, energy production, and even emotional stability.

Food is biological instruction.

What we eat teaches the body how to respond.

Healing does not require perfection. It requires direction, patience, and repetition.

Occasional deviation does not undo progress. Chronic disregard does.

Small, consistent choices create deep change.

The body responds to what we do most often — not to what we do occasionally.

Chapter 19 — Therapeutic Nutrition During Crisis

There are only so many hours in a day and only so much space in the body.

During a serious health crisis, nutrition must become intentional. Every meal, every drink, and every supplement must serve a purpose.

The goal is not simply to eat more food or to gain weight.
The goal is to change the internal environment of the body.

During Manuel's illness I had three objectives guiding every decision about what he consumed:

- remove what burdens the body
- flood the body with nutrients
- introduce substances that help eliminate harmful organisms

Healing nutrition must accomplish all three.

At the same time calories still matter. A body fighting disease requires energy. But those calories must come from foods that support healing rather than burden detoxification systems.

Developing Manuel's intake required constant balance between nourishment, cleansing, and strategic therapeutic foods.

Asparagus

Asparagus became one of the foods I used very intentionally.

It is known for its detoxification and anti parasitic properties and has long been used in supportive cancer nutrition. It also supports kidney function and elimination. Asparagus is a nutrient-dense vegetable rich in vitamins A, C, E, and K, as well as folate and fiber.

It supports digestion, heart health, and cognitive function, and it acts as a natural diuretic that helps the body eliminate excess fluids and toxins.

Asparagus is also a source of **glutathione**, one of the body's most important antioxidants. Glutathione helps reduce inflammation and protects cells from oxidative damage.

Beyond simply serving it with meals, I prepared it in a more concentrated form.

I cooked asparagus lightly in water, blended it into a smooth puree, and stored it in a glass jar in the refrigerator. Manuel took one tablespoon three times per day before meals.

It was simple, but consistent.

Aloe Vera

Aloe vera is often referred to as a miracle plant because of its remarkably rich composition. It contains more than seventy active compounds, including vitamins, minerals, enzymes, amino acids, and beneficial plant polysaccharides.

One of the most important compounds in aloe is **acemannan**, which supports immune function and cellular communication.

Aloe is widely known for its ability to promote healing in the body, particularly in the digestive tract and skin.It helps calm inflammation, supports the gut lining, and has natural antibacterial and antifungal properties. For internal support we used **Stockton Aloe**, a high-quality brand known for preserving the natural activity of the plant.

He started slow with just 1oz 3 times a day but then went up to 4oz. The ideal I believe is 8 oz, but it is not easy to tolerate so we didn't push it. He felt definate help with digestion especially during chemo. Chemo tears the gut and anything you can find to soothe it is a win.

Amla

Amla, also known as Indian gooseberry, is typically consumed as a dried powder and is often added to smoothies or drinks.It is one of the richest natural sources of **vitamin C** and is considered a powerful antioxidant food. Amla supports immune function, helps protect cells from oxidative stress, and contributes to overall vitality. Because of its high nutrient density, it is widely regarded as a traditional superfood in Ayurvedic medicine.

Lemon and Garlic Paste

Another remedy I prepared was a mixture of lemons and garlic.

It was not pleasant — I will admit that openly — but it was powerful. Organic lemons were thoroughly washed and blended whole with the peel and seeds. Several cloves of garlic were added to the mixture and everything was blended into a paste.

The mixture was stored in a glass container in the refrigerator.

One tablespoon was taken two to three times daily and swallowed quickly, followed by water.

Lemon supports detoxification and mineral balance, while garlic has long been known for its antimicrobial and immune-supportive properties. Together they created a very strong cleansing combination.

Apricot Kernels and Vitamin B17

Apricot seeds are known for containing compounds often referred to as **vitamin B17**.

These compounds have been discussed for decades in alternative cancer research. While controversial in conventional medicine, many practitioners still use them cautiously as part of supportive protocols. Apricot kernels are extremely bitter and must be introduced slowly.

Manuel began with three seeds per day and gradually increased his intake over time. Eventually he was consuming up to twenty seeds per day, divided between morning and evening. They were not pleasant at first, but like many things in healing, the body eventually adapts.

Moringa and Wheatgrass

Certain plants are extraordinarily dense in nutrients and have been used in therapeutic nutrition for generations.

Two that we incorporated were **moringa** and **wheatgrass**.

Wheatgrass is a highly concentrated nutritional plant often referred to as a superfood. It contains chlorophyll, vitamins A, C, and E, iron, magnesium, amino acids, and many important enzymes. Wheatgrass supports detoxification.

Wheatgrass is often taken as a concentrated juice shot. Many people find the taste very intense, and Manuel was no exception.

For some people it is easier to tolerate when added to smoothies rather than taken alone.

Moringa leaves are known for containing a wide spectrum of vitamins, minerals, and antioxidants. In many parts of the world they are considered one of the most nutrient-dense plants available. There is even a theory that in extreme conditions a person could survive on very small amounts of moringa due to its nutritional density, though of course it would not provide sufficient calories. Moringa leaves contain high levels of iron, calcium, protein, vitamins A and E, and numerous antioxidants. Moringa helps reduce inflammation, supports blood sugar balance, and contributes to overall metabolic health. It is also known for supporting liver function and detoxification processes. Because of its nutritional density, moringa is often used as a powerful supplement during times when the body requires additional support. In a healing protocol, however, its value lies in providing concentrated micronutrients.

Juicing as a Daily Foundation

Fresh vegetable juice became one of the central pillars of Manuel's nutrition.

Juicing allows large quantities of vitamins, minerals, enzymes, and phytonutrients to enter the body quickly without placing heavy demands on digestion. Carrot juice was the primary foundation.

Carrot Juice

Fresh carrot juice became one of the foundations of Manuel's daily nutrition.

Carrots are rich in **carotenoids**, including beta-carotene, alpha-carotene, lutein, and zeaxanthin. These compounds function as antioxidants and help protect cells from oxidative damage. Carrots also contain unique plant compounds called **polyacetylenes**, which are known for their anti-inflammatory properties. Regular consumption of carrot juice helps support the immune system, nourish the body with vitamins and minerals, and provide easily absorbable nutrients during times when digestion is compromised. Carrots contain numerous beneficial compounds and have been widely used in supportive cancer nutrition. Over time Manuel drank enough carrot juice that even his naturally darker skin developed a slight orange tint. This is completely normal when large amounts of carrot juice are consumed consistently.

Black Seed Oil

Black seed oil is another traditional remedy used across many cultures.

Black seed oil comes from the seeds of **Nigella sativa**, also known as black cumin. It contains more than one hundred active compounds and has long been used in traditional medicine for its immune-supportive and antimicrobial properties. Black seed oil is known for its strong antifungal and antiparasitic activity and is often used to support the body during infections.

Its taste is extremely strong.

Manuel once described it as tasting like brake fluid that had splashed into his mouth while working on a car. That description stayed with me. He took it in liquid form, which is considered the most potent way to consume it. I personally could not tolerate the taste after hearing his comparison and chose to take it in capsules instead.

Turmeric

Turmeric is a powerful anti-inflammatory root widely used in both traditional medicine and modern nutritional practice. Its main active compound, **curcumin**, helps regulate inflammation and supports immune balance. Turmeric also contributes to healthy circulation and cellular protection.

We incorporated turmeric into everyday cooking whenever possible — in soups, rice dishes, beans, and many other meals — making it a regular part of the diet.

Boswellia (Frankincense)

Boswellia, also known as frankincense, is a resin traditionally used for its powerful anti-inflammatory properties. It supports immune function, joint health, and inflammatory balance in the body. Boswellia supplements are often used alongside turmeric because the two compounds complement each other well.

We also used **frankincense essential oil**, placing a small drop under the tongue or on the roof of the mouth. While strong in aroma, it has a surprisingly pleasant taste and was part of our daily routine.

Propolis

Propolis is a resin-like substance produced by bees to protect their hives from infection. It contains a rich combination of **flavonoids, phenolic acids, terpenes, vitamins, and minerals**, giving it strong antimicrobial and antioxidant properties.

Propolis supports immune function and helps the body defend against bacteria, viruses, and fungi. It is also known for its anti-inflammatory effects and is often used to support respiratory health and skin healing.

Therapeutic Teas

Teas provided a gentler way to introduce medicinal herbs into the body without creating the feeling of swallowing endless supplements.

I described earlier how I combined several herbs into what we called our **Healing Tea**.

Herbs such as sage, nettle, burdock root, dandelion, red clover, cat's claw, chamomile, peppermint, and corn silk provided anti-inflammatory, detoxifying, and immune-supportive properties.

Drinking these teas daily created a steady flow of beneficial plant compounds entering the body without overwhelming the digestive system.

Healing Tea Blend — Herb Benefits

Sage

Sage is a powerful medicinal herb traditionally used for its antimicrobial and antioxidant effects. It supports the immune system and helps reduce inflammation in the digestive tract and respiratory system. Sage also contains compounds that help protect cells from oxidative stress, which becomes particularly important during illness and recovery.

Nettle

Nettle is one of the most mineral-rich plants available. It contains iron, magnesium, calcium, potassium, and many trace minerals that support blood health and overall vitality. Nettle also supports kidney function, helps cleanse the blood, and is known for its anti-inflammatory properties.

Burdock Root

Burdock root has long been used in herbal medicine as a powerful blood purifier and detoxifying herb. It supports liver function, promotes elimination of toxins through the skin and kidneys, and contains antioxidants that help reduce inflammation in the body. Burdock is also commonly included in traditional cancer-support herbal formulas.

Dandelion

Often dismissed as a simple weed, dandelion is actually a potent medicinal plant. Both the root and leaves support liver detoxification and bile production, which helps the body process and eliminate toxins more efficiently. Dandelion also supports digestion and provides important minerals.

Red Clover

Red clover has traditionally been used to support lymphatic circulation and blood cleansing. It contains natural plant compounds called isoflavones, which have antioxidant properties. Herbalists often include red clover in formulas designed to support detoxification and immune balance.

Cat's Claw

Cat's claw is a rainforest vine known for its immune-modulating properties. It supports the body's natural defense mechanisms and has been studied for its anti-inflammatory and antioxidant effects. Many practitioners include it in protocols designed to support the immune system during chronic illness.

Corn Silk

Corn silk — the delicate fibers found inside corn husks — is surprisingly medicinal. It supports kidney and urinary tract health and acts as a gentle diuretic, helping the body eliminate excess fluids and toxins. It also has soothing anti-inflammatory properties.

Chamomile

Chamomile is well known for its calming effects on the nervous system. During illness and stress, it helps promote relaxation and supports better sleep. It also soothes the digestive tract and reduces inflammation, making it especially useful for individuals dealing with digestive sensitivity.

Peppermint

Peppermint supports digestion by relaxing the muscles of the digestive tract and improving bile flow. It helps relieve bloating, nausea, and stomach discomfort. Its refreshing flavor also made the tea blend much more enjoyable to drink regularly.

How We Used the Tea

I blended these herbs together in proportions that felt balanced and brewed them as a daily tea. Both Manuel and I drank it regularly. It became one of the easiest and most pleasant ways to support the body without feeling like we were constantly taking supplements.

Herbal teas may seem simple, but when used consistently they can deliver a steady supply of beneficial plant compounds that support detoxification, circulation, and immune health.

Essiac Tea

One tea deserves separate mention: **Essiac tea**.

Essiac is a well-known herbal formula traditionally used in supportive cancer care. It contains a specific combination of herbs designed to support detoxification and immune function.

Preparing Essiac requires patience. The herbs must be simmered for a specific period of time, allowed to steep for many hours, then strained and stored. It is usually brewed in large batches and consumed in measured portions throughout the day. For us, it became another consistent part of the routine. Healing rarely comes from one miracle remedy. More often it comes from many small actions repeated consistently over time.

Rebuilding the Gut Microbiome

Chemotherapy, antibiotics, stress, and illness can severely disrupt the gut microbiome.

The digestive tract is home to trillions of microorganisms that help regulate immunity, digestion, inflammation, and nutrient absorption.

When this ecosystem becomes imbalanced, digestion suffers and immune function can weaken.

Rebuilding the microbiome became another part of our strategy.

In addition to fermented foods, I began preparing homemade yogurt using carefully selected bacterial cultures.

These beneficial bacteria helped restore microbial balance and improved digestive comfort after chemotherapy sessions.

Supporting the gut meant supporting the immune system.

Vitamin C IV

High-dose intravenous vitamin C delivers vitamin C directly into the bloodstream, allowing much higher concentrations than oral supplements.

Vitamin C plays a key role in immune function, collagen production, and antioxidant protection. In high doses it helps reduce inflammation, protect cells from oxidative stress, and support the body during periods of illness.

Many people report improved energy levels, mental clarity, and overall well-being after vitamin C IV therapy. It has also been widely used as supportive care during cancer treatment to help reduce fatigue and improve quality of life.

Healing Together

While Manuel followed the protocol most strictly, I did many of these things alongside him.

Not to the same intensity — I was still caring for children, managing the household, and handling endless responsibilities — but I participated where I could.

Partly because I believed in the benefits.

And partly because I understood something else.

If disease is influenced by infections, parasites, toxins, and immune stress, then the environment around the patient matters as well.

And stress itself is powerful.

The level of stress I carried during those months was enormous. Supporting my own body was not only about health — it was about survival.

Healing became something we were doing together.

Chapter 20 — Parasites, Internal Terrain, and Hidden Burdens

When people think about disease, they often search for a single cause.

A virus.
A genetic mutation.
A bacterium.

But the body rarely operates through single causes. Chronic illness almost always develops through a combination of stressors — what I described earlier as a perfect storm.

Toxins, infections, chronic stress, nutritional deficiencies, environmental exposures, emotional strain, and immune exhaustion all interact with one another. Over time they change the internal terrain of the body.

Understanding that terrain became an important part of the strategy we used during Manuel's illness.

Internal Pollution Goes Beyond Toxins

When people hear the word pollution, they usually imagine chemicals in the air, contaminated water, pesticides, or heavy metals.

Those are real and important concerns. But internal pollution goes beyond chemical exposure.

The body also carries unprocessed emotional stress, unresolved experiences, chronic worry, and the constant stimulation of modern life. These invisible burdens affect the nervous system, immune function, hormone balance, and digestive processes.

The body does not clearly separate physical and emotional input. What is not processed is held, and what is held eventually affects function.

Over time these accumulated burdens weaken detoxification pathways and create conditions where disease can develop more easily.

A Silent Presence

Parasites are rarely discussed in modern medicine unless they produce dramatic symptoms. Yet many organisms live quietly in the body, drawing resources, irritating tissues, and interfering with normal digestive and immune function.

A single female roundworm, for example, can lay hundreds of thousands of eggs in a short period of time. Once conditions become favorable, populations can expand rapidly.

Cooking temperatures may destroy live parasites, but eggs can be far more resilient. When consumed, they may remain dormant for years — sometimes decades — waiting for the right internal conditions to activate.

Immune Stress and Activation

The immune system plays a crucial role in keeping parasitic activity under control. As long as immune function remains strong and the internal environment remains balanced, many organisms stay inactive. However, when immunity becomes compromised — through chronic stress, emotional overload, illness, exhaustion, or antibiotic use — dormant organisms may activate.

In such cases infestation does not necessarily occur because of new exposure, but because the internal terrain has changed. This helps explain why symptoms can sometimes appear suddenly, without an obvious external cause.

Antibiotics and Microbial Imbalance

Antibiotics can be lifesaving and are sometimes necessary. But they do not discriminate between harmful and beneficial organisms. Their use disrupts protective intestinal flora, weakening one of the body's most important defense systems.

In this altered environment, parasites, yeast, and pathogenic bacteria can gain an opportunity to proliferate. Balance does not automatically restore itself once medication is stopped. The digestive ecosystem often requires intentional rebuilding through diet, probiotics, and cleansing protocols.

How Parasites Enter the Body

Parasites are present throughout the environment and can enter the body through many pathways:

- improperly washed or undercooked food
- contaminated water
- airborne particles and dust
- soil exposure
- insects and animals
- household pets
- shared surfaces and close contact

• travel and environmental exposure

Modern hygiene reduces these pathways but does not eliminate them.

Where Parasites Thrive

Approximately ninety percent of parasites affecting humans reside in the gastrointestinal tract, particularly the small intestine where nutrients are abundant. Others may inhabit various tissues, including the liver, lungs, muscles, joints, blood, skin, and even the nervous system.

They thrive in environments that are:

• toxic
• inflamed
• nutritionally imbalanced
• immunologically weakened

In other words, they flourish when the internal terrain becomes compromised.

How Parasites Burden the Body

Parasitic organisms can affect the body in several ways.

They may:

• release metabolic waste and toxins into the bloodstream
• damage intestinal lining and digestive tissues
• trigger inflammatory and allergic responses
• consume vitamins, minerals, enzymes, and nutrients
• weaken immune defenses

The results may appear in many different forms: fatigue, digestive disturbances, skin problems, allergies, mood imbalance, nutrient deficiencies, cravings, and chronic inflammatory conditions. These symptoms are often treated individually without addressing the underlying imbalance that allowed the organisms to thrive.

Parasites and the Cancer Question

During my years of studying holistic medicine, I encountered many theories about the relationship between infections, parasites, and cancer.

One of the most controversial voices in this area was Hulda Clark. Through years of microscopic research she proposed that many tumors contained parasitic organisms and that eliminating these organisms could influence disease processes.

Whether one agrees fully with her conclusions or not, her work raised an important question:

What role do hidden infections and toxic environments play in chronic disease?

Many microorganisms commonly carried by humans have been linked in research to long-term tissue damage and increased cancer risk.

Examples include:

• Helicobacter pylori, associated with stomach ulcers and certain gastric cancers
• Epstein–Barr virus, which affects immune cells and has been linked to several cancers

• herpes viruses, which remain dormant in many individuals and may reactivate during immune stress
• fungal overgrowth such as Candida

These organisms are surprisingly common.

In fact, many tests do not determine whether someone has been exposed — they measure antibody levels to determine whether the organism is active or dormant.

This raises an important question.

If many people carry these organisms, why do some develop disease while others remain healthy?

The answer often returns to terrain.

Immune strength, detoxification capacity, nutritional status, and overall internal balance determine how the body responds.

Two people may encounter the same toxin or microorganism, yet their bodies respond very differently.

The Question That Troubled Me

For years I considered the possibility that tumors might contain parasitic components. If that were true, the strategy would be straightforward: remove the parasites and cleanse the terrain.

But Manuel's illness presented a different puzzle.

He had lymphoma — a cancer of the blood and lymphatic system.

There was no solid tumor to attack.

So the question became much more complicated.

If the disease existed within the blood and immune system itself, how do we address that terrain?

At the time we approached the problem from every possible angle — cleansing, strengthening immunity, improving nutrition, reducing toxic load, and supporting the body in every way we could.

Years later I came across research by a Soviet-era professor who studied the organism Trichomonas and its potential role in blood disorders and cancers.
Trichomonas is best known for causing urinary infections, yet it is extremely resilient and capable of surviving in different tissues. It can be transmitted through water, shared surfaces, and even swimming pools, where chlorine does not always eliminate it completely.

One of the simplest natural substances long known to inhibit its activity is something most people would not expect.

Cranberry.

For many years I had already used cranberry juice and cranberry extracts successfully in treating recurrent urinary infections.

Seeing that connection again reminded me how often simple natural tools can support the body in ways that modern medicine sometimes overlooks.

The Invisible Chemical Burden

When people begin thinking about detoxification, they usually focus on food.

But food is only one part of the chemical burden the body carries.

Modern life exposes us to thousands of synthetic compounds every day — many of them quietly entering the body through pathways we rarely consider.

The skin absorbs.
The lungs absorb.
Even simple household contact introduces chemicals into the bloodstream.

The body does not evaluate these exposures separately. Every substance must be processed through the same detoxification systems — primarily the liver, kidneys, lymphatic system, and digestive tract.

Over time, the accumulation of these substances increases the body's toxic workload and can contribute to inflammation, immune stress, and metabolic imbalance.

Understanding these hidden exposures is an important part of reducing the burden placed on the body.

Cookware and Kitchen Toxins

The kitchen should be a place where food supports health. Yet many common cooking materials introduce chemicals directly into meals.

Non-stick cookware coated with compounds such as Teflon and other PFAS chemicals can release toxic particles when heated, especially when the surface becomes scratched or overheated. These compounds have been studied for their persistence in the body and their potential effects on hormone regulation, immune function, and liver health.

Plastic containers present another concern. When heated — especially in microwaves — plastics can release substances such as phthalates and bisphenols, chemicals known to interfere with endocrine signaling.

For this reason many practitioners recommend preparing food using more stable materials such as:

- stainless steel
- cast iron
- glass
- ceramic

These materials do not leach synthetic chemicals into food during normal cooking.

Personal Care Products

Another significant source of chemical exposure comes from products applied directly to the body.

Skin absorbs a large portion of what touches it.

Cosmetics, lotions, deodorants, shampoos, and other personal care products often contain dozens of synthetic ingredients designed to preserve, scent, or stabilize the product.
Common additives include:

• synthetic fragrances
• parabens
• phthalates
• formaldehyde-releasing preservatives
• petroleum derivatives

Many of these compounds were developed for shelf stability rather than biological compatibility.

Because these products are applied daily, small exposures accumulate over time. The skin becomes another pathway through which chemicals enter the bloodstream.

The same principle applies to nail products, hair dyes, and certain salon treatments, many of which release vapors that are inhaled as well as absorbed through the skin.

Air and Inhalation Exposure

The lungs represent one of the most efficient absorption surfaces in the body.

Anything inhaled enters the bloodstream quickly.

Household products often release volatile compounds into indoor air.

Examples include:

• air fresheners
• scented candles
• aerosol sprays
• cleaning products
• synthetic fragrances

These products may create pleasant scents, but they frequently release chemical mixtures that the body must detoxify.

Even small exposures repeated daily add to the body's cumulative toxic load.

Why Reducing Toxic Load Matters

When toxins accumulate in the body, they do more than burden detoxification organs.

They change the terrain.

The internal environment of the body — the balance of minerals, oxygen levels, immune strength, microbial balance, and the efficiency of elimination — determines what kinds of organisms can survive and thrive inside us.

In a clean, well-functioning environment, the body keeps most microorganisms under control.

But when the terrain becomes overloaded — through chemical exposure, poor nutrition, chronic stress, infections, and metabolic congestion — the balance shifts.

Inflammation rises.
Oxygen delivery may decline.
Immune defenses weaken.
Waste begins to accumulate in tissues.

These conditions create an environment where opportunistic organisms can flourish.

The body has remarkable detoxification systems designed to protect us.

The liver transforms toxins into forms that can be eliminated.
The kidneys filter the blood.
The lymphatic system removes waste from tissues.
The digestive system carries toxins out of the body.
The lungs eliminate volatile waste though breathing.

But these systems have limits.

When the incoming burden exceeds the body's ability to process it, toxins begin to accumulate.

Healing is not only about what we add to the body — nutrition, supplements, treatments.

It is also about what we remove.

Chapter 21 — Supplement Strategy and Rotations

As soon as we received the call confirming that something serious was happening, the shock lasted only a short time before action began. We began immediately — doing what I knew how to do.

Knowing that many chronic diseases are associated with toxicity, microbial imbalance, and parasitic burden, I decided to start with what I already knew well from my practice: cleansing and antimicrobial support.

The goal at that stage was simple — throw everything reasonable at the problem while we were still waiting for more precise medical information.

Reducing Microbial Burden (Parasite Support)

The first protocol we began was Hulda Clark's parasite cleanse, which includes three herbs:

- Black Walnut Hull
- Wormwood
- Clove

These herbs are traditionally used together because they target different stages of the parasitic life cycle.

Black walnut hull helps address adult organisms, wormwood supports elimination of intestinal parasites, and clove targets parasite eggs that can otherwise survive and re-hatch.

I specifically chose Hulda Clark's protocol because I trusted the integrity of her work. I had met her personally and had followed her research for many years. In my experience, the quality of her formulations was far superior to most commercial blends.

Many supplement companies combine these herbs into a single capsule. While convenient, this approach often reduces the potency and flexibility of dosing. In practice, these herbs work best when taken separately and according to a structured protocol.

Additional Antimicrobial Support

Alongside the parasite protocol, I added several natural compounds known for their antimicrobial activity.

Grapefruit Seed Extract

Grapefruit seed extract has strong antifungal and antibacterial properties and is often used to help control yeast and microbial overgrowth in the digestive tract.

Cranberry and D-Mannose

Cranberry and D-mannose are widely used for urinary tract health. They help prevent harmful bacteria from attaching to the walls of the urinary tract and support the body's ability to flush them out.

At this stage, the diagnosis was not yet confirmed. I had also not yet encountered later research suggesting that certain infections may play a role in blood cancers.

Looking back, I am grateful that cranberry and D-mannose were part of the early protocol because they are also known to support the body in managing Trichomonas infections, which some researchers believe may contribute to inflammatory conditions and blood cancers.

Adjusting the Strategy During Chemotherapy

Once Manuel entered the hospital and chemotherapy began, my focus shifted.

At that stage parasites were no longer my primary concern. Chemotherapy is designed to destroy rapidly dividing cells, and it does not discriminate between harmful and beneficial cells.

In other words, it kills a great deal of everything.

The challenge during chemotherapy is not only surviving the treatment but helping the body recover afterward.

Healthy cells must rebuild. The immune system must recover. The digestive system and microbiome must be restored.

This is where nutrition, juicing, and targeted supplements became essential.

Core Nutritional and Cellular Support

Liposomal Vitamin C

High doses of vitamin C are widely known for their antioxidant properties and their ability to support immune function. While Manuel received intravenous vitamin C once per week, he also took liposomal vitamin C daily, typically at doses several times higher than standard recommendations. Liposomal delivery improves absorption and allows vitamin C to circulate in the bloodstream more effectively than many traditional oral supplements.

Selenium

Selenium is an essential trace mineral that plays a key role in antioxidant defense and immune regulation. It supports enzymes involved in protecting cells from oxidative stress and contributes to thyroid function and metabolic balance.

Vitamin D with K2

Vitamin D plays an important role in immune system regulation, bone health, and inflammation control. Because vitamin D works closely with calcium metabolism, it is often paired with vitamin K2, which helps guide calcium into bones rather than soft tissues. Together they support immune function and overall metabolic health.

Bosmeric-SR (Boswellia + Curcumin)

Bosmeric-SR is a combination of boswellia (frankincense) and curcumin (turmeric extract). Both compounds are widely known for their powerful anti-inflammatory effects. They support joint health, immune balance, and cellular protection. The combination provides stronger anti-inflammatory support than either compound alone.

Proteolytic Enzymes

Proteolytic enzymes break down proteins. Unlike digestive enzymes, which are taken with meals, proteolytic enzymes are taken on an empty stomach. In that environment they circulate in the bloodstream and help break down inflammatory proteins and cellular debris. They are often used in protocols designed to support immune function and reduce inflammation.

Probiotics

Because chemotherapy and antibiotics can severely disrupt the gut microbiome, probiotics became essential. Healthy intestinal bacteria play a crucial role in digestion, immune function, and nutrient absorption. Rebuilding the microbiome was a key part of restoring overall health.

IP-6 (Inositol Hexaphosphate)

IP-6 is a naturally occurring compound found in many plant foods, especially grains and seeds. It is often used as a supplement to support immune function, cellular health, and antioxidant protection.

Maitake D-Fraction

Maitake mushrooms contain compounds that support immune activity.

The D-fraction extract is a concentrated form of these compounds and is commonly used to support immune system balance.

Manuel typically took about twenty drops three times per day.

Berberine

Berberine is a plant compound found in several medicinal herbs. It supports blood sugar regulation, gut health, and antimicrobial balance. It is also commonly used in protocols targeting microbial overgrowth.

Quercetin

Quercetin is a plant flavonoid found in many fruits and vegetables. It functions as a powerful antioxidant and helps regulate inflammation and immune response. Quercetin also supports respiratory health and cellular protection.

Rotation and Balance

At any given time Manuel was taking roughly ten supplements, which I rotated every couple of weeks with another group of supplements.

The purpose of rotation was to avoid overwhelming the body and to maintain effectiveness. When the same compounds are used continuously, the body may adapt and their impact may diminish.

By rotating supplements, we were able to provide broad support without excessive burden.

Healing is rarely about one miracle compound. More often it is the result of many small actions working together over time.

Chapter 22 — The Nervous System, Emotions, and the Body's Ability to Heal

From the beginning, I approached Manuel's illness the only way I knew how — holistically.

As a practitioner, I had spent years observing how the body functions as a single system. Nutrition, detoxification, immune function, emotional state, and even spiritual outlook are deeply connected. Treating only one aspect rarely produces lasting results.

So while we focused heavily on diet, supplements, cleansing, and therapies, I was always aware of something equally important: the state of the nervous system.

The nervous system regulates nearly every process in the body. Digestion, detoxification, immune activity, hormone balance, circulation, and tissue repair are all influenced by it. When the nervous system is balanced, the body can direct its energy toward healing. When it is overwhelmed, the body prioritizes survival instead.

Serious illness can easily push the nervous system into a prolonged state of alert. Fear, uncertainty, hospital environments, and the pressure of life-changing decisions all contribute to this. When that state continues for long periods, digestion weakens, inflammation increases, sleep becomes shallow, and the body struggles to repair itself efficiently.

The body is not malfunctioning in this situation.
It is protecting itself. For healing to occur, the nervous system must periodically shift out of survival mode and into a state where restoration becomes possible. This is where emotional states begin to matter just as much as physical treatments.

Acute Stress vs. Chronic Stress

Not all stress is harmful.

Acute stress is the body's natural response to an immediate challenge. In these moments the nervous system releases adrenaline and other stress hormones that sharpen focus and mobilize energy. Heart rate rises, muscles prepare for action, and awareness becomes heightened.

In short bursts, this response is protective and necessary.
The problem arises when stress stops being temporary.

Chronic stress occurs when the body remains under continuous pressure for long periods of time — emotional strain, financial uncertainty, responsibility, fear, or unresolved tension. The stress response never fully turns off. Stress hormones remain elevated and the nervous system becomes locked in a defensive pattern.

Over time this affects nearly every system in the body.
Many people living through serious illness experience this state for months or even years without realizing it.

Emotional Outlook and the Body

The mind constantly interprets the world around us, and the body responds to those interpretations.

When the dominant emotional state becomes negative — expecting the worst, focusing on danger, anticipating failure — the nervous system receives signals that reinforce stress.

This does not mean that negative emotions should be suppressed. Fear, grief, anger, and frustration are natural responses during difficult circumstances.

But when these emotions become constant, the body remains trapped in a heightened state of vigilance.

Healing requires moments where the nervous system experiences something different — safety, calm, connection, and hope.

Fear During Illness

Fear is one of the strongest signals the nervous system can receive.

In moments of fear the body prepares for danger. Stress hormones rise, muscles tighten, digestion slows, and immune responses shift. This response is useful when escaping immediate threats. But when fear becomes constant, the body remains locked in that defensive state.

Serious illness naturally brings fear with it — fear of death, fear of suffering, fear of making the wrong decision, fear of the unknown. Yet a body constantly preparing for danger cannot easily focus on restoration.
This is why emotional reassurance, faith, and belief become so important during illness. They are not abstract comforts. They are biological signals that survival is still possible. When the nervous system senses possibility instead of doom, the body responds differently.

Hope and Belief

Hope is often dismissed as something purely emotional, but biologically it carries real influence.

When a person believes that healing is possible, the body continues investing energy in repair. When a person believes that the outcome is already decided, the nervous system begins to withdraw effort.

Hope alone does not cure disease.

But hope changes the environment in which healing takes place. During Manuel's illness we intentionally surrounded ourselves with messages of possibility. Affirmations, prayer, meditation, and conversations about recovery all reinforced the same direction — that life was still moving forward.
Hope became part of the treatment environment.

Forgiveness and Emotional Release

Forgiveness is often misunderstood.

It does not mean approving harmful actions or pretending painful experiences never occurred. Forgiveness simply means releasing the emotional weight of carrying resentment indefinitely.

Holding anger or resentment keeps the nervous system activated. The body remains tense, and the mind repeatedly revisits the same emotional injury.

When forgiveness occurs, even partially, the nervous system can begin to relax. Many people experience a physical sense of relief when they finally release emotional burdens they have carried for years.

Letting go does not erase the past.

It simply frees the body from continuing to relive it.

Gratitude and Emotional Regulation

Gratitude may appear simple, but its effect on the nervous system is powerful.

When attention shifts toward appreciation — for life, for support, for small moments of beauty — breathing slows, muscles relax, and stress responses decrease.

Gratitude does not deny hardship. It simply allows the mind to recognize that even in difficult circumstances something meaningful still exists. This shift creates physiological changes. The nervous system moves away from constant vigilance and toward balance.

Practices That Supported Us

During Manuel's illness I intentionally introduced practices that could help stabilize the nervous system.

Affirmations and breath work became part of our daily routine — simple tools that helped calm the nervous system and support the body while everything else was unfolding.
None of these practices replaced nutrition, therapy, or medical treatment. But they supported something equally important — the internal environment in which healing was taking place.

The Caregiver's Nervous System

Serious illness does not affect only the patient.

Caregivers often carry an enormous emotional and physiological burden. They become decision makers, organizers, researchers, emotional stabilizers, and constant observers of the patient's condition.

What people don't see is that the caregiver never leaves the situation. Even when the body rests, the mind keeps scanning — symptoms, decisions, what's next. There is no off switch. Just a constant low hum of responsibility.

Looking back, I now realize that while Manuel's body was fighting lymphoma, my body was carrying the weight of responsibility. Every decision felt critical. Every symptom mattered. Every appointment required attention.

At the time there was simply no space to process it.

The body keeps track of these things quietly.

Sometimes the effects appear later, long after the immediate crisis has passed.

Why Emotional Health Is Often Ignored

Modern medicine focuses primarily on physical interventions — surgery, medication, radiation, measurable laboratory values.

These tools are incredibly valuable and often life-saving.

But the emotional environment in which healing occurs is rarely addressed with the same seriousness. Stress, fear, hopelessness, and emotional exhaustion can significantly influence biological processes, yet they are often treated as secondary concerns.

Holistic approaches recognize that emotional regulation is not a luxury during illness.

It is part of the healing system itself.

When emotional balance improves, digestion improves. Sleep improves. Immune responses stabilize.

The body begins working with treatment instead of struggling against constant stress signals.

Healing Happens in the Whole System

Over time I became even more convinced of something I had already seen many times in practice.

Healing is not one intervention.
It is the result of many systems working together — body, mind, environment, and belief.

When the body feels safe enough to shift out of survival mode, it begins to access its natural ability to heal.

Chapter 23 — The Life After

During the battle there is no time to feel.

There is only time to act.

Decisions must be made quickly. Information must be gathered. Treatments must be arranged. The next step must always be taken before the mind has time to wander too far into fear.

The body enters a strange state during crisis. It runs on purpose and adrenaline. Exhaustion exists, but it is ignored. Emotions are pushed aside because there is simply no space for them.

Survival becomes the only objective.

Looking back now, I realize that those years were lived in exactly that state.

We fought.
We researched.
We prayed — not out of routine, but because there were moments when nothing else reached that deep.

We juiced vegetables at midnight and drove to treatments at sunrise. We counted supplements, measured drops, blended herbs, and studied protocols. Every day had a mission.

There was no time to collapse.

And somehow, through all of that, Manuel survived.

But something few people talk about happens after the battle ends.

The silence arrives.

The hospital visits stop. The tests become less frequent. The emergency energy that carried you through the crisis slowly fades.

And suddenly the body begins to feel what it never had time to feel before.

For many survivors and caregivers, the true processing of the experience begins only after the danger has passed.

The nervous system, which had been locked in survival mode for so long, finally begins to release its tension.

Sometimes that release appears as exhaustion.

Sometimes it appears as emotional overwhelm.

And sometimes it appears physically in the body.

In my case, it appeared in my back.

At the time I did not fully connect the two. I only knew that pain arrived suddenly and intensely. Sitting became nearly impossible. Sleep became difficult. My body felt as if it had been carrying something heavy for too long.

Only later did I understand what had happened. The body had been holding what I didn't have time to feel.

For years I had carried responsibility without pause. Decisions about treatments, nutrition, finances, family, and survival all rested on my shoulders.

I carried it willingly. There was no other option.

But the body remembers what the mind pushes aside.

When the war ended, my body finally set the weight down.

In the middle of crisis, everything feels immediate and absolute. Every decision carries enormous weight. Every symptom feels like a message that must be interpreted.

But distance brings clarity.

Looking back now, there are several things I understand more deeply than I did then.

First, healing is rarely the result of a single intervention.

Medicine helped Manuel survive. Chemotherapy reduced the immediate danger. But nutrition, cleansing, emotional support, faith, and the daily work of rebuilding his body all played their part.

The body does not heal through one system alone.

It heals when many systems begin working together.

Second, fear is powerful — but belief is powerful too.
Fear narrows the mind. It convinces the nervous system that danger is permanent. When that happens the body struggles to access its restorative functions.

Hope, faith, and determination create a different environment. They remind the nervous system that life is still possible.

Third, caregivers carry their own invisible battle.

When someone is diagnosed with a life-threatening illness, attention naturally focuses on the patient. But behind every patient there is often someone else holding the structure of daily life together.

That person becomes the organizer, the researcher, the emotional stabilizer, and often the decision maker.

The weight of that role is rarely acknowledged.

Yet it is real.

And finally, illness changes people.

It changes relationships, priorities, and the way time is experienced.

Some things that once seemed important lose their meaning completely. Other things — quiet moments, simple conversations, laughter around a dinner table — suddenly feel far more valuable than they ever did before.

Survival rearranges perspective.

Five years have passed now.

Manuel is alive.

Life is not exactly the same as it was before lymphoma entered our home, but perhaps that is not the goal.

Some battles change everything.

They change the way you see time, the way you see people, the way you see your own strength.

We learned things we never expected to learn.

We discovered strength we did not know we had.

And we saw, very clearly, how fragile and precious life really is.

The war ended.

But healing, in many ways, continues.

If you are reading this because someone you love has heard the word cancer, know this:

The moment of diagnosis feels like the end of the world.

But it is also the beginning of a fight — one that may reveal a strength you didn't know you had.

You may discover courage you did not know you possessed.

You may discover resilience hidden deep within the body.

And you may discover that healing is not a single decision or treatment.

It is a process that involves the body, the mind, the people who stand beside you, and the belief that life is still worth fighting for.

The tools may come from medicine, from nature, or from faith.

But it all comes down to the quiet determination to LIVE.

Mindset creates the will to live.

Purpose fuels that will.

Support strengthens the body.

And survival only matters if we learn how to live again.

About the Author

Elena Rybak is a holistic health practitioner with more than twenty years of experience supporting clients through nutrition, detoxification, and lifestyle-based healing approaches. Her work focuses on helping the body restore balance through diet, cleansing, and nervous system support.

Her understanding of integrative healing deepened further when her husband was diagnosed with aggressive lymphoma in 2021. The experience led her to combine conventional medical treatment with intensive nutritional and holistic support strategies, many of which are described in this book.

Elena is also the author of *When the Body Speaks* and the **Healthy Me!** series of children's books focused on nutrition and healthy habits.

She lives in Florida with her family.

More information about her work can be found at:
www.LivingHealthyInstitute.com

www.ingramcontent.com/pod-product-compliance
Lightning Source LLC
LaVergne TN
LVHW090524110826
845146LV00003B/968
9798995518006